LIFE MAPPING

DECODING THE BLUEPRINT OF YOUR SOUL

KAREN LOENSER

DEDICATION

I come from a long line of Seekers, who have relentlessly explored and exercised many modalities, tools and practices to help them understand the key milestones of their life's journey and find the meaning of their soul's purpose.

I am so grateful to my mother Lo Anne and Grandmother Lois for being early pioneers and sharing their experiences, books and teachers that have inspired me to become an explorer of life.

I give thanks to all those who have walked with me along my life's path and shared opportunities for me to make choices between love and fear along the way. I recognize all of you for the powerful co-creators you are, and that we chose this together long before we were born.

Most of all, I send all my gratitude to my soul- team, Ralph, Lauren and Graham. My children are far wiser that I will ever be, and my husband, the keeper and protector of my heart, is quite literally, the better half of my soul. I love you for your faith and encouragement, and all you have sacrificed to help me follow my dreams.

Lastly, but from my heart, this book is for you dear reader. As you go through these pages, I wish for you to find and recognize the roots of your purpose. For you to seek and find the true meaning that you have intended for your own "earth school" experience. May you find the light that will spark your own inner seeds to grow as you map your own life's path forward.

Let's go forth and explore it together!

Not until we are lost
do we begin to
understand ourselves.

Henry David Thoreau

CONTENTS

SECTION ONE:
WHERE YOU'VE BEEN: YOUR
LIFEMAPPING JOURNEY SO FAR...

SECTION TWO:
WHERE YOU ARE: YOUR LIFEMAPPING
JOURNEY TODAY

SECTION THREE:
WHERE YOU ARE HEADED: YOUR
LIFEMAPPING PATH FORWARD...

> "THERE IS NO
> GREATER AGONY
> THAN BEARING AN
> UNTOLD STORY
> INSIDE YOU."
>
> MAYA ANGELOU

INTRODUCTION

THE BEGINNING: WELCOME TO YOUR LIFEMAP

I was in line for my morning coffee when I saw Pat. Slim, attractive, in her mid-fifties, she was then one of the few high-ranking women in our company. We had worked together only a few times, but I had coached her through some important employee town hall meetings, in my then role as an Executive Producer at AT&T. We bonded, as women do, when the pressure to step up and lead in the spotlight is at its highest, and she steadily rose in rank and respect alike, taking on each new challenge with grace. It had been weeks since I'd seen her and I was shocked by her appearance. She looked frail and exhausted. Not at all like her confident, always-put-together self.

We sat down at a quiet table in the corner of our office cafeteria, and she told me that her husband had moved out and filed for divorce. "I know it sounds like a cliché," she said, idly stirring her coffee, "but I swear, I never saw it coming."

She talked about the garage sale, the agony of the legalities, of cancelling their upcoming anniversary trip to Italy. Her son was away at college. Her daughter was living a few states away with infant twins and a busy job. She didn't want to burden them with her sadness.

My heart went out to her as she described the sudden betrayal and feeling of the road dropping out from under her. "Where do I go from here?" she asked, clearly at a loss for answers.

I felt a surge of guilt, as I inwardly judged her situation. Clearly, she'd been working too much, trying so hard to climb the corporate ladder, that she let her relationships slide at home.

"The funny, thing is," she continued, as if reading my mind. "I never really wanted this job. And now it's all I have."

As we finished our coffee, she said goodbye with one sentence that I'll never forget.

"Life, they say, is what happens when you're busy making other plans."

It felt like a warning.

The words hung in the air between us for a long moment. Was that an old Beatles song? The ending to a sad movie? It felt empty and defeated, like a tale about a life imagined but never lived. A mask with an unseen soul underneath.

I gave Barbara a hug for strength and made a vow that would never be me.

When It Happens to You

Fast forward the time machine ten years later. Exactly two months before my 50th birthday, I woke up certain that my life was over.

It was a Thursday morning. I could hear the distant sound of my alarm going off. For one beautiful moment I forgot where I was.

But in the next instant, the all too familiar feeling of regret and sadness rushed over me in a drowning wave of shame. I remembered how I got there. And most of it had nothing to do with the bottle of Chardonnay I drank the night before.

I shut off the alarm, yearning for the mind-numbing sleep to return so I could avoid another day. To escape that morning after reflection of my dull disappointed eyes looking back at me in the mirror.

On paper, it was my prime time. My daughter was in college and my son was in middle school. The days of carpools and teenage mayhem were mostly over. I was crossing over the bridge to "me" time. I felt like I was finally growing up.

We'd moved to Dallas less than a year before to a beautiful house in the suburbs. It was our first year of southern living, after taking a corporate relocation package that moved our family from New Jersey to what we'd hoped were new adventures in the warm and welcoming south. We were excited about the opportunity to start over in a new place, with new friends and a less hectic pace of life.

I also embraced this change to begin a new chapter in my career. I had landed a promotion in a newly created role in my company, where I could start applying my experience in television and advertising. I was eager to work on exciting new projects that would expand our corporate brand.

I had a new team, and felt my professional confidence and inspiration finally taking hold.

I was also, for the first time, taking care of myself. I had carved out a mindfulness practice. I was meditating and journaling. I was running five miles a day. I was eating well and feeling good. I was tuned in, tapped in and turned on.

It was all perfect. Until it wasn't.

I was nine months into the new job when I was informed that a new director had been brought on board to "support" some of my expanding job responsibilities. The new hire was a former colleague of my boss from her previous job who she thought could bring "new perspective" to the role.

My role. My promotion. My hard work...that had earned me the title, the team, the glass door office. Without a word, or discussion, it was snatched out of my hands and handed over to someone else.

I was humiliated, confused and angry. I'd been a career renegade all my life. I had worked extra hard for everything I got. Clearly, the team-up had been planned from the minute my boss even came on board. But on that day, I was sentenced by the judge of "not enough." And it crushed me.

But here's the thing.

It would be months before I would understand this...but it wasn't really me who took the fall. It was my ego. In my heart, I knew that even though the job looked amazing on paper, it was fraught with flaws. Like a VP who inflicted his own fear of failure onto his team. A department of competitive infighting that only manifested distrust. Daily fire drills with no defined purpose or goals. We all had beautiful titles, but it was at the price of selling our souls.

When I could finally step back about all my self-disappointment, doubt and fear, I realized that I hated that job. It was wasting my time, talent and all that was authentically me.

And my soul was slowly dying.

But I didn't realize all that at first. Instead, I did what I always did. I blamed myself. I played my "not enough" record, that allowed my ranting ego to restate my failure over and over again. I was flawed and a fraud. I would never be successful. And, perhaps worst, I felt too old and defeated to start over again.

Until that moment, I thought I was the solo pilot of my life. In charge of the direction...captain of my flight plan. But after every take-off, there was another crash landing... onto another runway in a place that I didn't want to be.

In reality, I knew that I was on autopilot. And I had no idea where I was going. And then I remembered Pat's haunting words. "Life is what happens when you are busy making other plans."

How the hell did I get here?

As so, on that June morning, 60 days before my 50th birthday, as I lay there in my bed, I let go. And the road I was on fell away from me.

Through my bloodshot eyes, under those blankets, I started thinking about all of the milestones that had led me to this crash...plotting through all of the memories that had gotten me to that place of feeling like my life was a failure.

One by one, they replayed like a movie in my mind. Complete with the people, the emotions. The decisions, and the consequences. The Love and the Fear. And finally... the Impact. And the Meaning.

And that changed everything.

Creating the Life Review Before the Review

As I sped down the highway towards my mid-life defining moment, I skidded off the roadway onto a completely uncharted and unpaved road. It was the road to my passion. It was the road to my heart story. It was the road to everything that was authentically me.

And that, as they say, has made all the difference.

That pivot gave me the map back to my soul. And I can help you chart yours.

I'm offering you the opportunity to take your life's journey to a whole new place. A place you may never have imagined. To understand the blueprint of you; a blueprint that you may never have thought possible. And the best part is that I'm offering you the "map" on how to get there. Your soul map. And you were born with it.

How Do I Know? Oh, My Friend, Because I Wrote the Book on It. And It's in Your Hands!

The idea of life mapping came to me through the desperation and lowest point of my own experience. As I take you through the process of deciphering your own life's map, I'll share my story...and stories of others who have used this simple practice to uncover their own life's path.

None of them are famous. They've become self-change makers who have used this tool to shift their path. Consequently, they are living the life, experiences and lessons *they planned before they were born.*

Life can be what happens as we're making other plans. And I also believe that the past *holds the keys to helping* you shape and re-define your future. And it all begins by recognizing the choices we make between *love* and *fear.*

Yeah, two words that can lead us completely towards or away from our soul's planned purpose. And we come here wired with our own inner guidance to help remind us along the way.

These next few chapters will help you utilize your past milestones to have a clear and inspiring path to your future.

And we'll get you there in a way that is easy, inspirational and fun.

Finding the Meaning in Your Milestones

If you're questioning your life's choices up until now, I'll help you decipher the clues to show where you are already fulfilling your life's purpose. And from this place of inspiration, you'll be able to define your plan – and understand **what you came to do.**

We'll also utilize simple, fun and trackable tools to help you understand your own unique skills and talents to map out **where you're going.**

Learn what you can do right now at the present moment to take control of your journey. Use this as a tool to release blame, fear or guilt from the past.

Take a moment to recognize the many important milestones of your path to understand your relationship with love and fear to plot your "Lifebeat" towards the experiences your soul intended.

The reward? You will recognize every experience and person as an opportunity for your soul to learn, grow and evolve. And most important of all, none of life is just happenstance. You are divinely guided and have chosen this life with all its experiences for your soul's growth and a very specific purpose.

This book is for you if...

- You're at a major crossroad in your life, like a divorce, job loss or a health scare
- You have kids who are ready to leave the nest or perhaps you are single and feel disconnected or unsure of what to do next.
- You 're living with anxiety, depression or loneliness.
- You're ready to release blame, fear or guilt from the past.
- You want to know what you can do right now to take control of your journey.
- You've made up your mind that you don't want to waste any unnecessary time discovering your life's purpose.

This book will show you the meaning behind why you're here, where your talents lie, why you've experienced what you have and what you can do to live the life you were born to live.

Get ready to be amazed.

I'm here to tell you that there is a compass, a Lifemap, that will reveal the blueprint of your soul. If you spend a little time with this book, it will show you the way.

Time to Get Off Your "But's"

I'm also here to tell you that you are NOT alone. When I had the courage to share my story, I was amazed by the number of people that said they felt the exact same way. Similar to how I used to feel, they felt like they were wearing a mask while editing a script and the perfect image just to showcase their well lived life on their Facebook page. And all along, they defied the truth of themselves. They denied their heart.

There are a million excuses for staying put and I've tried all of them.

Here are the top 3 big ones:

1. **But**, I just don't have time. (You can read this book in less than 3 hours).
2. **But**, I'm too old. (Vera Wang, Lucille Ball, Martha Stewart, Julia Child, Ronald Reagan, Morgan Freeman, Viola Davis – launched their careers in midlife).
3. **But,** I don't know what I want to do. (Ah, it's there, in your heart, waiting to be uncovered. That's why you're here with this book in your hands)

We have all been there. And we've all felt overwhelmed. I know what it's like to get to a place on the journey and feel like too much time has passed to make a change – to shift old habits, reshape a new body, a new mind, a new perspective. To begin again. **To make new plans.**

How does that saying go? *A journey of a thousand miles begins with a single step.* And I promise, these steps of the soul mapping process will lead you on that journey.

We all have a purpose and a story to tell.

Let's go discover yours.

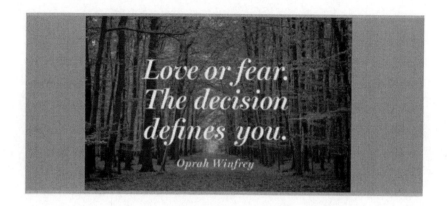

Love or fear.
The decision
defines you.

Oprah Winfrey

CHAPTER 1

WHAT'S A LIFE MAP?

How I Got Here

I like to tell people that I grew up in a "metaphysically religious" household.

It's a self-made description, meaning I'm a "mixed breed" of spiritual dogmas. Half-Roman Catholic and half Spirit Seeker – two divine ideologies threaded together by a soul.

And while both have shaped my journey and the life I've led, I can now see that none of it was by accident.

My spiritual matriarchs, without a doubt, are my mother and grandmother, who were both avid believers in the God of the Church and the Spirit of the metaphysical. While they were well respected in the pew, they were also consumers of all the New Age books that were coming out in the late 70's and early 80's. I read all of them, and particularly loved the ones that talked about past lives and channeling higher spirits. It just seemed an extension of what the angels and the saints stood for, but without all the rules.

Lo Anne, the mother of me and my five siblings, was at her core, a textbook Catholic. She read "The Lives of the Saints" to us at the dinner table and led the Friday night family rosary as we all perched on our skinny knees on pillows in front of the statue of the Blessed Mother. She even had the Archbishop of New York on speed dial.

Further indoctrinating my religious DNA, were my father's two brothers, who were Benedictine Monks. You know the kind that wear brown robes and live in a monastery? Do not be fooled. They were a bad-ass band of brethren, with fiery, "holier than thou" stubborn attitudes, who showed up regularly, usually with their priestly entourage, unannounced at our dinner table.

So yeah, we were *that* kind of Catholic family. And it was pretty great.

But just to spice up my spiritual curiosity, I would also come home after school some afternoons, only to discover psychic mediums, energy healers and astrologers engaged in deep conversation with my mother in our kitchen. When Maya showed up, she'd park her RV in our driveway, which was packed to the rim with ancient books, crystals, candles and her pet cats. If you look up the word Gypsy, Maya's face would be there, complete with the wiry hair, bangled bracelets and flowing skirts that smelled like sage. She was magical and I swear could both read and predict your every thought.

Maya said she could read the multi-dimensional energy co-existing with us under our rooftop. She identified the spirits of two lost Indian children living in our basement and recounted her own past life romance as my father's royal mistress when they lived together in Atlantis.

One of Maya's best moments was when she took on my Benedictine uncles at a dinner debate over the legitimacy of astrology. The monks decreed it a blasphemous parlors game set up to dupe people's obsession with knowing their fortunes. But Maya, in her all-knowing, mystical voice, recounted in vivid detail the glorious pilgrimage of the magi astrologers who were not only priests and kings themselves but also had the foresight to follow a star and be the first to find and welcome baby Jesus in the nativity.

Did they think it just a coincidence that the Christ Child was welcomed first into the world by the three Magi or wise men, as they came to be known? While the Priests and Rabbi's overlooked the event living their lavish lifestyles in their castles, and in doing so, overlooked the most important coming in the history of the planet? I mean what can you say after that? Dumbfounding silence is what happens. I saw it. Maya smiled, snapped and dropped the mic on those brethren know-it-alls, and I loved her.

It was around this same time in my early teenage years that my mom gave me an audio recording of a reading of my birth chart by Clare Houston, who was then a world-renowned British astrologer. She had done my reading, along with my other siblings, as a gift from, who else, my Grandmother. I was mesmerized by how Clare was able to recount every aspiration that I inwardly felt of what I wanted my life to be but had never shared with anyone. Given only my name, birthdate and the time and place where I was born, she was able to tell me every detail about my talents, desires, and personality. It was if she could magically peer into a crystal ball and see everything in my potential future. She assured me in her aristocratic drawl, that the stars held a vast portfolio of talent and opportunities ahead. A "Me" that I could not remotely fathom as a then shy, skinny 13-year-old with braces. I came alive in that moment of Clare's proclamation of my potential. It was if she had tapped into my deepest, most personal wishes and dreams. Like a fairy godmother, she unleashed all my possibilities with a wave of her magic wand.

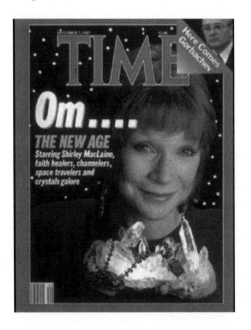

After that, I devoured every metaphysical book I could find. The infamous astrologer, Linda Goodman's book "Sun Signs" brought the entire astrological calendar to life, profiling every sign of the zodiac with her outrageously theatrical and poetic flair. Jonathan Livingston Seagull portrayed the mystical and metaphorical story of the afterlife through the tender story of a rebellious seagull. "Seth Speaks" introduced a series of conversations with a channeled spiritual guide on the other side. Edgar Casey, known as the "Sleeping Prophet" offered thousands of readings about Atlantis, reincarnation, and energy healing.

And then, in the mid-eighties, "Shirley McClain's" Out on a Limb" launched a book, a movie, and a tabloid revolution that took meditation and channeling guides and spirits out of the closet onto the front page of Time Magazine. The date was February 7, 1987 and the New Age had begun.

By the mid-nineties, Oprah began interviewing some of these metaphysical "up and comers" on daytime television. I remember racing home from work to try to grab the tail end of her conversations as these fascinating writers and visionaries shared their stories, many for the first time, to audiences that for the most part, had no idea what they were talking about. But for me, it was my language, I found my people and I hung on to every word with one "aha!" moment after another.

It was around that time that Gary Zukav's "Seat of the Soul" and Marianne Williamsons "Return to Love," were brought to the national stage by Oprah. It was Oprah's quest for asking life's biggest questions, that woke millions up with the idea that we are indeed all souls seeking our life's purpose.

Her show was all about telling those stories. It became my place for spiritual exploration. For me, this forum offered me the people and the conversations that became a wakeup call for my heart, mind and spirit. And from that day on, I knew I needed to understand *why* I was here.

These were the teachers that introduced me to what the soul really is. It's not, as I was taught, a virtual scorecard of sins and good deeds that lives invisibly in your chest and carries the record of all our good and bad deeds. And it's certainly not finite and limited to this lifetime. In the Oprah classroom, I learned that I am an individual soul with a consciousness that never really dies, that comes to this "earth school" over and over again for a variety of experiences.

Oprah's platform equipped me with a deep understanding of my ever evolving and temporarily human version of "me." A perfect, limitless soul with eternal, ever-changing potential. Unlike anything I had ever learned in a church pew, that was what made me feel like a real spark of God.

And so are you.

Your Life by Design

So that was just a little bit about me for your context. Most of the time you invest in these pages, is going to be purely about you. Your journey to unravel your own lifemap. The book in your hands will help you find the blueprint for rediscovering your life's purpose.

I believe we all map out a plan for our lives before we make the decision to head down to this planet. We are, as they say, "spiritual beings having a human experience," and we carry within us a plan for what we want to accomplish in each lifetime. These plans are our own unique "soul maps" which chart the course of the experiences we intend to have in each lifetime.

I like to think of our soul map as our imbedded lesson plans that are specifically designed by our "higher selves" and our spiritual guides to promote our soul's growth and development. The purpose of us coming to our "earth school" is far from random. It's our soul's desire to immerse ourselves with other humans to share experiences that will help us evolve into higher beings of light and love. This, in its simplest terms, is the meaning of life.

With the help of our many angels and guides, w
an intricate plan for what we want to learn. Perh
path to learn more about forgiveness, faith or self-love.
Some call this karma, which many people misunderstand. It's
not a punishment for what we have done in past lifetimes,
but more of an opportunity to go through experiences
that allow us to love more fully. This becomes part of the
blueprint of your soul map.

While we are in between lives, we see our life experiences very differently. We can objectively view all of our
past mistakes and failures from the perspective of our
true essence, which is pure love. Like a parent, looking at
their child from a place of limitless understanding, we too
can see our true selves and the driving force behind all
our decisions. We are able to access the choices that we
made in each lifetime and determine if they came from a
place of love or fear. So, rather than coming from a place
of judgement standing in our earthly shoes, we see only
our soul's essence trying to navigate through our chosen
pathway with an inner compass of love or fear.

This emotional dance is what you do with your heart, with
every person that you meet, every decision that you make
– it's the pendulum of your emotional compass tracking the
"life-beat" of your soul. It's a GPS. A compass. The basis of
all experiences. Your Milestone maker. And this is where
you will learn how to read its guidance for you.

Your Soul Team

We never come into any of our lives alone. Instead, we
come into this lifetime with a personally chosen squad of
supporters who are here to assist us on our life's journey.

As we make our plans for what we want to learn in each lifetime, we enlist the help of other souls to join us on the journey. And all of these soul connections join our journey from a place of pure love. You often choose to incarnate with those you've been with through multiple lifetimes. I like to call them your "soul squad." And together you formulate a plan for how you can integrate and interweave the intentions each of you have for your own life's journey.

If, for example, you've planned an opportunity in this lifetime to learn more about the lesson of forgiveness, you may set up a plan with a difficult mother-in-law or an unfaithful husband. Or you might choose instead to supersize that lesson by experiencing an even more difficult opportunity to put forgiveness into practice: like how to heal through a broken heart and forgive the drunk driver who killed your son, or an abuser who took away your childhood.

With our earth consciousness, it is hard to imagine that we would ever "choose" these kinds of terrible experiences, and that the people who may have harmed you the most, could be part of your beloved soul group. But every person who comes into our lives and plays an emotional role (either positively or negatively) has, in fact, made a divine agreement with you. These souls have chosen to play a "spiritual" role in your life with the intention of offering you an opportunity to make a choice; to learn more about love.

I like to imagine this is like being the writer, producer, director and actor in the movie of your life with a marquis of actors in roles you've specifically chosen and cast. It puts a bit of a different spin on your nasty neighbors, bossy bosses, and exasperating exes, doesn't it? In this version of life, you can view everyone who has had any kind of influence on you as a teacher with a powerful lesson, instead of an arbitrary or inflicted part of your life's experience.

Unfortunately, part of the lesson of coming to life school and creating our life movie, is that we forget all of this before we are born. It's part of the soul's journey to not remember the intention, but instead, learn about it through our inner compass and life's experiences. We must rely on our hearts to navigate it all. To remember what we have forgotten.

And this, my friend, is how life-mapping works.

Here's how this book breaks down:

Sometimes, the biggest hurdle to starting off on any real quest is trying to see the big picture and breaking down the steps it takes to get there. When I started anything, even as a kid, I had to map out a plan. I had to start with the macro to get to the micro.

When I was in college, long before the days of fake news, my journalism teacher taught us the best way to tell any story was to break it down from the perspective of the 5 W's – the who, what, when, where, and why. So, that's how we're going to break down the soul map of your life.

Each chapter is designed to break out your life story around the 5 W's in a really simple way.

SECTION 1.
WHERE YOU'VE BEEN: YOUR LIFEMAPPING PAST

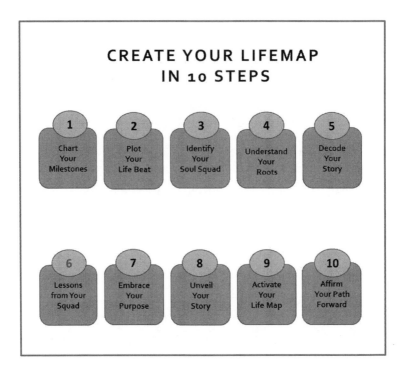

Chapters 2 through 7 will lay the foundation of your soul story. In these chapters we will explore your **PAST** – here's the breakdown.

1. **Chart your milestones** will take you through your "**WHERE's**"- the places, the experiences, the actions and activities of your life. Here you will look at the top 20 milestones in your life and lay them out for the foundation of your Lifemapping story.

2. **Plot your lifebeat** will show you how to sketch out your "**WHEN's**" - when you made the choices,

decisions and preferences between love and fear and the outcome of those decisions along your path. Here you will review each milestone on your Lifemap and ask your heart the most important life question: "Did this experience teach me love or fear?"

3. **Identify your soul squad** will provide you with your "**WHO's**" - the key people and influencers in your life (big and small) and the roles they have played in your lifetime so far. These will identify your top 20 teachers of love or fear...these will reveal the people who have signed up to be your soul guides.

4. **Understand your roots** will help you understand your "**WHAT's**" and layer the early circumstances, situations and surroundings in your early life. As you came to understand the world, things like religion, poverty, politics, and world events influenced your opinions, beliefs and impressions of where and how you lived. This became the foundation of your love and fear compass... and your understanding of the planet. Here you will fill in the Lifemapping layers of how the world you lived in influenced your love and fear belief system.

5. **Decode your story** will have you dig into the big questions as you explore your "**WHY's**" – it's here you will begin to lay out the wholistic look at your life's purpose and how it plays out to give you the map of your life. It's compiling the "where", "when", "who", and "what" to see how they all fit together. This is where you will learn what your love and fear

milestones mean from the vantage point of your soul's purpose.

6. **Lessons from your squad** will help you identify who the key people have been in your life so far, and pin-point the ways your **"HOW's"** have impacted your life's path. Like Decoding your Milestone story, this is where you'll discover the life lessons your soul guides have come on this journey to teach you.

SECTION 2.
WHERE YOU ARE: YOUR LIFEMAPPING PRESENT

Chapters 8 & 9 - Once you've clearly laid out the past, now you must stand in the truth of your "now"- **YOUR PRESENT**- and map out how to take to your life's adventure path from here. This is a map to your future that you will chart and following it will lead to the manifestation of all you are meant to be.

1. **Embracing Your Purpose** will help you stand in your truth, savor the now and the recognition of who you have come to be. This is the place where we will savor the essence of the present moment where all our power is. This Lifemapping Layer will begin to help you fill in the colors of the map of you, by highlighting your talents and interests, your inner GPS that points your soul's north star.

2. **Unveiling your Story**– This is where you will define the meaning in your map by pulling your life story into one unified view of the amazing, impactful,

meaningful you. This is where the life review becomes the life renew...where you get to see the beautiful, self-actualized and self-orchestrated map of your soul. This is where you can step back to really see the tapestry of your life and how those threads have woven the fabric of who you are, and what you have come here to offer the world. This is where you will put into action ideas and exercises to release fear and set intentions for your lifemap from here.

SECTION 3.
WHERE YOU'RE HEADED: YOUR LIFEMAPPING FUTURE

And finally, with a clear understanding of your past and your purpose, and anchored fully in the present, we can embark on creating your vision for the future.

1. **Activate Your LifeMap** - This is where the magic happens...where your map reveals its story...this is where we take the incredible work you've done in the previous chapter's, and create the vision of your lifemap in one cohesive view. This is where you will learn the manifestation formula, for making your dreams come true!

2. **Defining Your Path Forward** – This is where we will tally up all of our strengths and self-truth's to create the vision of everything you want to do, be and have in the next phase of your life. Here you will learn how to articulate and define your purpose using powerful words that will create a positively charged vision

statement that is personally customized to your life and dreams.

3. **Your Soul Toolbox: Making Your Vision Come True** – This final takeaway chapter offers you tools to continue to acquire and inspire your ongoing growth, change and innovation as you continue down your path. Since we are "never done" our dreams will continue to bring us more opportunity to become ever more of what we've intended. This is where you learn how to continually recalibrate to "follow your bliss" to keep you in the "positive receiving mode" of your dreams while utilizing powerful tools of inspiration, intuition, intention and imagination.

How to Use this Book:

I've structured this book to offer more than just a "how-to" for creating your LifeMap. I also wanted to share inspiring quotes, mantra's and affirmations as well as stories, tools and practices from people who have influenced me along the way.

Soulfirmations - These affirmations will ground you as you go through each Lifemapping step. They are designed to be **3-minute inspirations and mantras** that can be practiced effortlessly, even if meditation or affirmations have never worked for you in the past.

	Life Mappers Stories- These are stories about real people who have utilized these practices in their lives to decode their life's purpose. These people have agreed to share snippets of their Lifemapping experiences and stories to help inspire you!
	Seeker Stories- I've been so incredibly fortunate to meet the most incredible soul-seekers along my journey…their stories will inspire you as they share moments when´facing their biggest fears showed them their life's purpose.
Lifemapping Exploration	**Lifemapping Explorations –** These are the step by step "how- to's" in each chapter that will help reveal the vision of your soul's purpose. Each is designed to be a fascinating adventure into your past, present or future self. These explorations will help you see the "you's" that you have been, the "you" that you currently are and the future "you's" will come to be.
	Soul Goody Bag: "Tools you Can Use" at the end of each chapter, that will include links to websites, audiobooks and videos. We put these within easy reach of each chapter so you can feel free to jump to a deeper level of understanding of the authors or teachers that inspire you, right as that "aha" hits you. Following that thread means that you are acting on that inspiration. I want you to pay attention to the thread and freely respond to it throughout this book. The more you engage, the more you will gain from this book!

That's a lot of information...so let's take a moment to breathe into our first Soulfirmation to launch the beginning of our journey. This is a combination of an affirmation and a meditative exercise that will ground you before we begin each exercise.

When you are ready to begin, repeat the following affirmation

This will take you no more than three minute's.

SOULFIRMATION #1

Close your eyes. Take a deep breath and picture the light of love surrounding you.

It encircles you in safety, in appreciation, in oneness.

See that light permeating your heart and your solar plexus, filling you with the bright pink glow of love and protection.

Appreciate this feeling of peace, openness and unfolding.

Sit with the light and continue to let it shine from within.

That, my dear friend, is what the light of your soul looks like.

Repeat the following Soulfirmation three times– continuing to fill yourself with light and love.

 SOULFIRMATION #1

"I am tuned in to the truth of my inner compass
and know I am on the right path
to discover, explore and embrace my soul's purpose.
I see the light. I know I am light.
I am willing. I am open. I am love. I am free.
I am ready to begin."

When you've finished the mantra, take a moment to breathe in and out slowly, sending gratitude back to your inner light.

So good. You have begun.

SOUL GOODY BAG

Here are some resources mentioned in this chapter for you for further exploration:

- **Linda Goodman's Sun Signs** - *Linda Goodman's Sun Signs* was published in 1968. This was the first astrology book ever to earn a spot on *The New York Times* Best Seller list.[1] It was followed by *Linda Goodman's Love Signs* (1978), which also made *The New York Times* Best Seller list and set an industry record with $2.3 million being paid for the paperback rights.

- **Jonathan Livingston Sea Gull** - written by Richard Bach and illustrated by Russell Munson, is a fable in novella form about a seagull who is trying to learn about life and flight. It is also a homily about self-perfection. Bach wrote it as a series of short stories that were published in *Flying* magazine in the late 1960s. It was first published in book form in 1970, and by the end of 1972 over a million copies were in print.

- **Seth Speaks** - The **Seth Material** is a collection of writing dictated by Jane Roberts to her husband from late 1963 until her death in 1984. Roberts claimed the words were spoken by a discarnate entity named Seth. The material is regarded as one of the cornerstones of New Age philosophy, and was instrumental in bringing the idea of channeling to a broad public audience.

- **The Sleeping Prophet** – by Jess Stern. Edgar Cayce was an American clairvoyant whose channeling sessions happened in a trance state where he would answer questions on subjects as varied as healing, reincarnation, dreams, the afterlife, past life, nutrition. Atlantis and future events. Cayce founded a nonprofit organization, the Association for Research and Enlightenment, to store and facilitate the study of his channelings.

- **Out On a Limb** - is an autobiographical book written by actress and dancer Shirley MacLaine in 1983. It details MacLaine's journeys through New Age spirituality. The book follows her from southern California to various locations including New York City, Europe, and Hawaii, culminating in a life-changing trip to the Andes Mountains in Peru. The book received both acclaim and criticism for its candor in dealing with such topics as reincarnation, meditation, mediumship (trance-channeling) and even UFO's

- **Seat of the Soul** – by Gary Zukav - *The Seat of the Soul* encourages you to become the authority in your own life. It will change the way you see the world, interact with other people, and understand your own actions and motivation. Beginning in 1998, Gary appeared more than 30 times on *The Oprah Winfrey Show* to discuss transformation in human consciousness concepts presented in this book.

- **Return To Love** by Marianne Williamson contains her reflections on the book *A Course in Miracles* and her thoughts on finding inner peace through love. In it is perhaps her most famous quote and her challenge at looking at our inner fears. "Our deepest fear," she writes, "is not that we are inadequate. Our deepest fear is that we are powerful beyond measure. It is our light, not our darkness that most frightens us."

SECTION ONE

WHERE YOU'VE BEEN: YOUR LIFEMAPPING JOURNEY SO FAR...

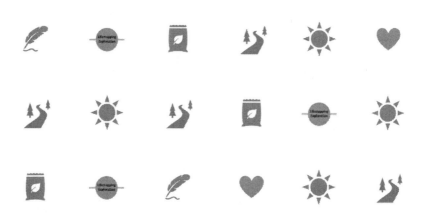

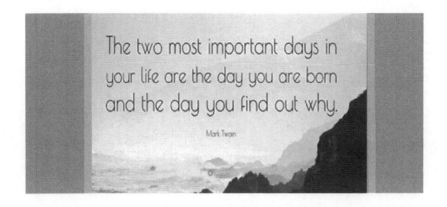

The two most important days in your life are the day you are born and the day you find out why.

Mark Twain

CHAPTER 2

CHARTING YOUR MILESTONES

How the Milestones Were Born

The day I lay in my bed a few months before my fiftieth birthday was a turning point in the way that I looked at life. It began with a flurry and fury of self-accusation, yelling at myself for the failure I had become, the life I wasted, the self I had let down.

It was in that darkest moment with the feeling of suffocating lack that if felt myself stop breathing. It was as if time, like me, was frozen...barren...*paralyzed.*

Through the tears of grieving the me I thought I was *supposed* to be, I came to realize everything I really was.

In my mind, a myriad of memories, milestones, milli-moments, all began playing out before my eyes. Like a kaleidoscope of intertwined snippets from the past, these visions began lighting up like fast frames in a slide show. It was a decoupage of images from my past, flashing with every blink of my eyes. In the beginning, they were random images, and then slowly, a pattern emerged.

I started plotting out all of the things that happened to me from birth up until the present moment. My metaphysical/religious childhood. My first marriage. The birth of my daughter. My divorce. Being a single mom. Remarrying. A near death experience during the birth of my son...it all slowly replayed before my eyes, like the life-review they say you experience after you die.

But I was still alive.

And maybe, just maybe, if I looked carefully, there might be purpose to it all?

I dragged myself out of bed and found a pad of yellow Post-it notes. On each piece of paper, I wrote down those significant moments of my life...getting married, giving birth to my daughter, getting divorced, getting remarried, giving birth to my son. My son's cancer diagnosis, my sister's suicide. One by one, the notes lined up in an unfolding story across my bedroom wall. And the picture of my life slowly unfolded.

It was a tale of failures and successes. Hope and abandon. Loneliness and completeness. Failing and resurrecting. Unraveling and rediscovering. Like the dance of waves, ebbing and flowing on to shore, through each layer of experience, each significant moment, the good and the bad...a tapestry of heart woven threads...the fabric of me, and my life.

And as I stepped back and looked, something beautiful came to light; it was the biggest revelation of all. Everything, every experience, every event, every circumstance, was a decision between love or fear. Each and every one.

As I traced each milestone, from one to another, a story emerged. A story of strength. A story of perseverance. A story of purpose. A story that took a lifetime to learn and a moment to decode. A story that brought me to the present moment.

With still approximately four more feet of totally open wall to decide what to post on my Post-it's next.

It was at that moment I asked myself a really important question. What did I want the rest of my story to be? What were the milestones that I wanted to see up on those Post-it notes?

And this is when I took my power back.

I decided that I would really, really go for it. From that point forward, I decided to embrace love and give fate a kick in the ass.

And this was the point that I did a pivot on the physical self and started my work on my soul self. I meditated. I journaled. I had conversations with myself. I began to look within. And that's when everything changed.

In the chapters that follow, I'll share how that morning changed me. But I will also show you how that day taught me that I wasn't a failure. That I already had achieved so much, I was just measuring myself by the wrong measuring stick. I was seeking self-love in all the wrong places. And it was hidden in the dark of ego and fear.

After that, it was no holds barred. I ran the Boston Marathon. I met my spiritual hero, Wayne Dyer. I landed a dream job at Discovery. I crafted the vision of "Mind, Body, Spirit" network. I personally pitched it to Oprah.

This is just a snapshot of my journey. And it began with understanding what my life's milestones had shown me, which gave me the courage to move forward in the clear direction of my dreams.

William Thoreau said it best over a century ago:

"Go confidently in the direction of your dreams! Live the life you've imagined." That was just an old saying until I understood it was the magic formula for living.

In the chapters that follow, I will give you play-by-play examples of how I whittled the process and shaped it into Lifemapping.

And I'll also be real with you about how I fell down. How I scrapped my knees (ego) and still yelled at God (a lot).

But I got up. I held fast to each milestone. I carried them. And then they carried me.

In this chapter you will:

1. Create Your Physical and Mental Space – to find the right materials and location for your Lifemapping.
2. Set Your Intention – with a calming mantra before you begin.
3. Chart Your Milestones – I will also share mine as a guide.
4. Journal Your Insights – with some questions to help jiggle the aha's.

All you have to do now, is say yes.

This is the experience that will provide you with the first important clues about those really important places on your life-map…. your **"WHERE's"**-where your feet and decisions have taken you: the places, the experiences, the moments, the actions and activities of your life. Your path up to now.

Are you ready?

Let's do this!! (And I'll be with you every step of the way.)

LIFEMAPPING EXPLORATION #1

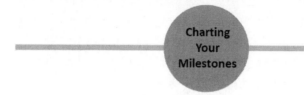

STEP 1: SELECT YOUR MATERIALS AND LOCATION

Prep-work is the rich soil into which great accomplishments (intentions) are planted.

(I'm not sure if that's a real saying, but you can quote me on that.)

The set-up in the life-mapping process is key to getting your mind and heart primed for the exercise.

And here's the best part...there's no real "technique" you need to learn or follow. Just like your life, you can create your lifemap however you want. If you want to get started right away, I suggest you start simply as I did with a pad of post-it notes, a sketch pad, a notebook or a blank sheet of paper. If you are feeling artistic, you can use colored markers, pencils, stickers or crayons. Many have enjoyed a whiteboard and a set of colorful dry erase markers. And, of course, you can also plot your milestones out on your computer, or even in the notes section of your phone.

This really is all about how you like to work and how to best capture your thoughts easily and effortlessly, as they unfold.

If you prefer creating a tangible (hard copy) version of your map, erase-able colored pencils or moveable stickers are also great materials especially if you want to design or draw your map on paper.

If you decide to do your map with Post-it's on a wall, you'll want a large, preferably private area, so you can leave your map up for a while. The Post-it notes is my favorite approach if you have a good place for it, as it will allow you to move the milestones around or squeeze in ones that you might not initially remember. It's also great to be able to leave it up in a place where you can look at it often, as it can ultimately become a vision board. (more on that later.)

The bottom line is that your technique is up to you. And If you want some ideas of other materials or approaches for your life map – I've posted a number of examples, including my own, on my website at www.KarenLoenserLifemapping.com

Once you've selected your mapping materials and have chosen your location, you can set the mood of your space with quiet mediation music, soft lighting or a lit candle, and a comfortable place to sit for reflection.

If you decide you want to Lifemap with a friend or part-ners, you'll want to allow for space for each of you to initially work separately, and then a table or group space, to share your experiences and observations, if you choose.

Lastly, if you have a notebook, keep it close by to log any thoughts, observations or feelings that come to you when you complete the first layer of your lifemap. I suggest a dedicated journal for this experience, as a lot of memories, emotions and observations will emerge.

STEP 2: QUIET YOUR MIND, CENTER YOUR SOUL, OPEN YOUR HEART

Once you have selected your space and haven chosen your mapping materials, the next important step is to take a few minutes to ground. Part of releasing fear and reaching out to love, is going within to where our "source" lives. "Grounding" means taking a moment to quiet your mind, center your soul and open your heart, so its voice can be heard. This doesn't have to take the form of a formal meditation process (although it can if you are comfortable with meditating). Grounding is mostly giving yourself some space to just breathe. It's a brief, dedicated moment just for you... like a moment of silence, or a dedicated pause.

This process can be as long as you want, but I suggest 2-3 minutes to allow yourself to quiet your thoughts so you can fully immerse yourself into the milestone mapping mindset. If this is hard for you, just try focusing on your breathing... deep inhale in...slow exhale out.

As you go through your grounding, remember to call in your higher self, angels, guides (or whatever spiritual power you are comfortable with) to be with you through this exercise.

No matter which form of grounding you choose to align your inner self before your milestone exercise, don't be afraid to call upon your *higher self* for inspiration. Your higher self is part of your inner knowing, the soul of you that fully remembers and understands your life's purpose.

STEP 3: SETTING YOUR INTENTION

Now that you have spent some time silently centering, you are ready to set your intention. This is a positive affirmation that will help bring clarity to what you want to learn and understand through your milestones. Intention will activate and energize your focus on bringing the best information from your higher self, so that divine insights will come to you through this experience.

Oprah set the bar, on the power of intention. It's widely known that no one could ever walk into a meeting, pitch a project or idea, without being able to articulate the intention of why they were doing it, and what they'd hoped to achieve for the end result. Intention is also about stating how you want to feel as a result of the outcome.

Here's an example of actionable intentions:

- My intention with this Lifemapping experience is to receive insights and guidance that will help give me clear ideas for the next steps I need to take in my life.
- My intention is to use this exercise to get to know what I love and what makes me happy, and to help me define and release what I don't love and what makes me fearful.
- I intend to be open and honest with the feelings that come from reviewing my life experiences, and no matter what, honor them for what they have taught me.

Asking is the gateway of activating and receiving. Ask for your most important milestone memories to come to you. Ask that they come to you easily and effortlessly. And ask that you are giving the most important information and ideas you need to fully unlock keys to your life's purpose.

Having intention is a great way to really put fear in the back seat. It puts you in charge of steering in the direction you want to go; in the direction of your highest good.

And so, dear friend, as you take this first step on your journey to discover your life's purpose, let's build you up with your next Soul – affirming thought:

SOULFIRMATION #2

"I am the creator of my reality.
I am grateful for all of the rich life experiences
that my soul has signed up for in this lifetime.
I am safe, protected, grounded and connected.
I embrace my life mapping journey from a place of readiness;
I am ready to learn about my soul's purpose and what it has to teach me."

Repeat the Soufirmation 3 times– continuing to fill yourself with light and love.

When you've finished the mantra, take a moment to breathe in and out slowly, sending gratitude back to your inner light.

And now, you are ready for your lifemap to begin to reveal itself to you.

STEP 4 CHARTING YOUR MILESTONES

I found the easiest way to "start the chart" is just to give a high-level "think" about your life's key moments.

Imagine you're meeting someone for the first time, and giving them an overview of your life resume. The things you did or the events that impacted you... both the good and the not so good happenings along your path. These can be **major events** or **stand-out moments** that impacted you in a meaningful or memorable way.

Think of it as a slide show of memories replaying the most impactful experiences of your life." These could be key rites of passage: graduations, achievements, weddings, jobs, relationships or deaths. Or memory markers: a teacher who recognized your talent, a time when you did something you were really proud of, a day that taught you gratitude or remorse, or giving up something you loved. Moments that taught you something about yourself, winning or failing: running a marathon, getting fired from a job, falling in love, getting your heart broken, saving a life or someone saving yours.

There is not a defined format for this. You can go in chronological order, skip around, backtrack, and rearrange. Just let the memories bubble up like little corks on the water.

As you move through these memories of your life, you can add as many as you like. Try to be open to including those that brought as much LOVE (Connective/Affirming experiences) into your life as FEAR (Disconnected/Non-Affirming experiences). Both are equally important teachers and will provide incredible meaning as you do your "Life Review" later in this book.

To help inspire you, I've included an illustration of my lifemap below. It looks much nicer here in the book, because I've had lots of time to share and re-edit it for my workshops, but you can see how it creates a simple timeline of my life. Again, do your own thing, in whatever format speaks to you.

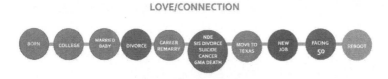

Suggestions for Going Through the Process:

1. **Give yourself a time limit.**
   Charting your milestones can take as little or as much time as It feels right to you, but I recommend giving yourself a time limit of no more than 20 minutes. Set a timer because it will help keep you on track.

2. **Try not to over-think it.**
   Memories are interesting things; they may begin in linear fashion but then you'll find all sorts of things may trigger other thoughts to come to the surface.

   And that's OK. But rather than letting that moment linger, just put the event on your timeline and move on to the next one. Try not to get too caught up in the details and the emotions attached to each milestone – you'll have time to go deeper later. Just think of this as a free association exercise that comes from your heart instead of your head.

3. **Try not to self-edit.**
   This may be the toughest part of the exercise. Just write whatever comes to you and don't be surprised if some of your milestones are seemingly less significant occurrences. You are looking for what comes to mind as "key moments." You may find a wedding or the loss of a parent may not come immediately to mind as a milestone. But the first time you went sailing, or wrote a poem, or read a certain book, came up as a significant event on your lifemap. Think of this as a free-association game and log whatever comes to mind first.

4. **Be gentle with yourself.**
   Some of this will come really easily to you...and some of this may trigger emotions and bring feelings to the surface that you don't expect, or that may surprise or upset you. That's ok....and totally normal. You're going back in time to an earlier "you." You may have forgotten some things...or even buried some stuff. We all do that.

5. **Don't worry about chronology:**
   You also don't have to look at this as a linear exercise. You may go right to your mid-life crisis, then back to your college rejection letter and, finally, to your first job promotion. The order of how the memories flow onto your lifemap doesn't matter, so freely chart them in whatever way they flow.

I found this coming up a lot in my workshops. Some folks stayed really high level on their chronological milestones while others dove hard and deep into their emotional back-stories. Here's the thing- you are letting your soul do the talking here. Let it be the boss. Let it remind you of all of the things that are important. Allow it to override that EGO driven head of yours for a bit. Let your heart be heard. Your happy heart, your broken heart, your confused heart. All of it.

Your heart will {IHEARTYOU} for it.

And when you do that, the really important things, the soul-voice of your purpose, will sing through because it won't focus so much on your life's resume. Instead, it'll hear the soul in your heart story.

LENA'S STORY: Reprioritizing Priorities

Lena admitted that she'd joined the Lifemapping Workshop because she wanted to "make some changes" in her life, but didn't know where to focus. She was a NYC pharmacist who had just been laid off and was in a relationship she felt was going nowhere. She seemed defeated, lost and just tired of the struggle of trying to "figure her life out."

When she got into the first part of the Lifemapping exercise, Lena was surprised at one of the first milestones that came up for her. It triggered something she'd suppressed for most of her life, and admitted it to our small workshop group for the first time.

From a very young age, Lena was able to hear and understand the thoughts and feelings of animals. She told the story of being eight years old, when her dog, Jasper, "told" her that he was dying. "He and I were very connected." she said, "I was an only child, and he was my dearest companion from the day I was born. I know it sounds weird, but I had whole conversations with him that I heard in my head. They seemed very real and normal to me."

Lena said at that age, she thought everyone could communicate with their pets, though she never talked about it with her parents.

"As I got older," Lena remembered, "I realized that "gift" I had made me weird, so I kept it to myself. But I have always been connected to animals and even to this day, I have a 6th sense about how they are feeling."

Lena was surprised when she listed that memory as the first milestone that came up. "I'd forgotten all about that connection to Jasper. But I remember the feeling of happiness that our relationship gave to me."

This is a great example of how the milestones that come up for you may not be in fact the more common occurrences like graduation or getting your driver's license. Instead, the really key milestones can be the ones that just come to you suddenly in your mind...the ones that have emotional impact tend to be the ones that are the most significant.

Lena went on to talk about how she had thought about becoming a vet, but had settled on a pharmaceutical degree since money was tight. It became a career that paid the bills versus giving her the connection she craved.

"I literally have a wall and a cash register between me and the patients that I am trying to help," Lena observed. "I never liked this feeling of being disconnected, which is why I think I always felt so unhappy in my job."

Lena's was a familiar story of how easily we can "settle" for less than what our soul intended. Her early connection with her dog was a vital life thread in her soul's tapestry...it was the beacon of "love" that was trying to signal her in the direction of her life's path. Second guessing that, even by taking a similar but less soul affirming step in the direction of our light is where our lifeboat can drift off course.

For Lena, it became clear that most of her early milestones connected to "Love", were associated with pets and her "gift" for understanding animals. As she reviewed her milestones, the "Love" came from her connection to her animal activities and relationships and the "Fear" came from her job, family expectations, her boyfriend, money and disconnection with her people relationships.

In reviewing Lena's milestones, it became clear that her connection to animals was part of her purpose, and gave her joy. And clearly, the juxtaposition of a so-called successful life as a pharmacist in the city, while making her appear "less weird" made her feel like an imposter.

So How Did Lifemapping Help?

Even though Lena lost her job and money was tight, she had time on her hands. So, we looked at things that could fill her heart, as well as her bank account. It wasn't about a full life transformation; it was about finding some "tweaks" that could open up a space to find ways to explore the places that fed her soul.

Lena was able to find a getaway spot for her a short train-ride out of the city where she could volunteer at a "half-way house" for abandoned horses. As often as she could, she would go out to the farm and work in the stalls. Eventually, it became her haven, and a place where her intuitive gifts flourished. In addition to the horses, she began to get to know the thoughts and feelings of the barn dogs, cats and even goats. Slowly, Lena was able to open up and share her gift of animal communication with the barn owners and vets, and began to find real validation to her intuitive skills. "Strangely, I'm not as good with the barn people," she laughed. Last we spoke, Lena had shifted out of her relationship, found a job closer to the barn still working as a pharmacist, but was also working on developing herbal remedies for animals. Lena is the perfect example of how we can all make subtle but powerful shifts from pain to purpose.

We are all born with this life purpose, but our life's work is to remember and live it. We all celebrate the day that we are born, but the real celebration does really come on the day we know why.

As you now step back and look at your own milestones from a holistic perspective, it would be a good time to grab your journal and reflect on a few questions. And as you do so, I would encourage you to try an experiment.

Try to take an objective step back and detach yourself from the personal experience of your story and look at your life from the perspective as if you were sitting in the audience at a theatre watching the unfolding of a movie of someone else's life, and not your own.

Imagine you are watching someone else's life story, without knowing all the details, or any of the emotions (as you do) behind each event.

 Ask Yourself:

1. How does your story feel when you look at it in the 3rd person?
2. Can you find empathy for the person who made the mistakes, or had the broken experiences?
3. Can you find admiration for your accomplishments, joys and triumphs?

I'm hoping that this will have you see a whole new vision of yourself, as I did. When I was able to sit in the "front row" of my own life, an amazing thing happened.

My own ego and self judgement went by the wayside. I was able to look at myself in a completely different way.

I saw determination. And vulnerability. And courage. And kindness.

I saw a person who tried very, very hard to do the right thing.

I saw a person who loved to be inspired and to inspire others.

I saw a person who was both blessed and also afflicted with hardship and adversity.

I saw a person that was loved for her spirit, as well as a person that did not always fit into the ego-driven corporate world.

I saw a person who was riddled with self-doubt who overcame great fear to do great things.

I began to really like that girl in a new way.

I began to be really proud of her

I began to believe she could do even bigger, greater things.

Let's try this on for you.

In the next chapter, we'll be taking a look at the meaning behind these milestones and how they reveal the clues to your life's purpose.

The key, as our friend Dr. Wayne Dyer loved to say, is to "Have a mind that is open to everything, and attached to nothing."

This is where the journey to true self-understanding begins.

> Love is what we
> were born with.
> Fear is what we
> learned here.
>
> Marianne Williamson

CHAPTER 3

PLOTTING YOUR LIFEBEAT

You still with me? If you made it this far, feel good about your progress!! These exercises are BIG, BIG, BIG!!

The journey of a thousand miles, they say, begins with a single step. And you've begun. Way to go! I'm proud of you!

Now that you have Charted your Milestones and have mapped out the foundation of WHERE you have been on your Lifemapping journey, this chapter will show you how to sketch out your **"WHEN's"**. By that, I mean that we'll take a look at when you made those choices, decisions and preferences between love and fear and the outcome those decisions had on your path.

The exercise is all about finding meaning in your milestones. And this next step for me, was the one that really brought my life's purpose to the surface.

This was the thing that got me out of my bed and back on track.

In this chapter, you will

1. **Plot Your Lifebeat** – and help define if that milestone moment was about love or fear.
2. **Explore the Emotional Scale** – our place of power that can help us evaluate our feelings, intentions and beliefs, and learn how reaching for a "thought that feels better" can impact our outcome.
3. **Calibrate Your Energy** – This is the force both within and with "out" your energy field that not only reflects your emotions but also your barometer on the "love and fear" scale. And yes, it impacts a lot of what you attract into your experiences. It's a "real thing" and we'll show you how you can control it.
4. **Create the Movie of Your Life** – We'll create the movie trailer of your life – and it won't feel weird, I promise.

Let me start with sharing mine.

My Lifemapping Movie:

OK, picture this, will you? I'm standing there in my bedroom, in my pajamas, with tear-stained, two-day old mascara on my face. Sobbing, as the Post-it movie of my life played out before me…literally, right before my blood-shot eyes.

Here's the movie trailer of how my milestone timeline played out:

Fade up on a scene from the early 1960's when the world was trying to recalibrate between love and war. Karen was born to a homemaker mom and a dentist Dad in the New Jersey suburbs and had a childhood full of love and lots of siblings. Her early years were enriched with fairy tales, doll houses and ballet lessons. Catholic school didn't ruin her but introduced her to the angels she could almost remember and nurtured her belief in unseen things.

Fast forward through girl scouts, and high school glee club. She dreamed of UCLA and California sunshine but settled instead on a woman's college in rural Missouri; her mother's alma matter. It was a cowardly choice, a safety school, but there, on that small, lonely, rural campus, she found and nurtured her life's true calling. To write and produce her own TV show. She wrote screen plays starring her in it, including writer, producer and director in the credits. She imagined the dress she'd wear to the awards show. Of course, no woman at the time was doing that, but she could feel it, the dream, the wish, the vision...ever so slowly, sprouting in her soul. Music up: Helen Reddy: "I am Woman, here me roar...." She could almost believe it.

Here the movie music changes from hopeful to melancholy. The scene darkens. Fear steps in, ridicules her dream and tells her that she's too small for such a big goal. Not smart-enough, pretty-enough, talented-enough, creative-enough...just not enough to have that vision...to imagine more than who she "really was." And she listens to the voice, not fully believing it, but still afraid to be seen or found out for the "not-enoughness" that she was.

The seedling in her soul wilts and fades. Karen opts for her next "safety move "and reaches towards a glimmer of love. She marries an illusion, a false promise of purpose.

But slowly, the truth fades through. This isn't Karen's dream, it was a delusion, a deviation. She was in a dance with the wrong partner. And deep inside she knew that the little seed of her life's true calling, was still slowly growing. The girl carries on, embracing a job at a tiny TV studio that loves her back and, soon after, a baby daughter who re-introduces her to wonder and joy and hope.

Scene changes... Husband leaves her for another woman. Karen scoops up her baby and goes back to her childhood home and becomes the very thing she most feared. A divorced, jobless, single mother. With the love of her family, she plots on...focused on her daughter and making ends meet. One decision, one moment, one day at a time.

And then, a crescendo. In the letting go, the joy comes in. Her hard work evolves into an amazing career. The seeds grow, success follows. Appreciation. Financial security flows. Karen stands in her light, and attracts a wonderful new partner, a man who loves her unconditionally. Another baby is on the way. The enough becomes abundance. The dream becomes reality.

And the happily ever after?

Again, fear steps in...the castle in the clouds crashing down.

Karen nearly dies in childbirth. But they reboot and recover. 9/11 changes the world forever. Six months later, their infant son is diagnosed with cancer. Her grandmother dies. Her sister goes through a traumatic divorce and commits suicide. Karen's once wonderful marriage starts to unravel. In a last-ditch effort to save it all, she and her family pack up and head for a new life in Dallas. But running from fear, only leads to fear. In their new beautiful home, her family is miserable. Then, her job promotion is ripped from her hands. She faces turning 50 and can't get out of bed.

See How I Did That?

Can you see the milestones? Love meets fear and fear meets love...then love meets fear... and fear meets love ... up, down. High, low. Like a heartbeat.

Here's a vison of what that looks like plotted out on a lifemap:

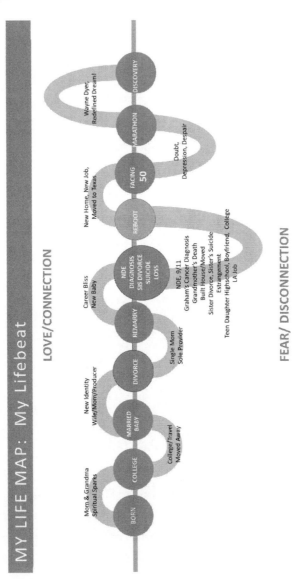

MY LIFE MAP: My Lifebeat

LOVE/CONNECTION

FEAR/ DISCONNECTION

BORN — Mom & Grandma Spiritual Sparks

COLLEGE — College/Travel Moved Away

MARRIED BABY — New Identity Wife/Mom/Producer

DIVORCE — Single Mom Sole Provider

REMARRY — Career Bliss New Baby

NDE DIAGNOSIS SIS DIVORCE SUICIDE LOSS — NDE, 9/11 Graham's Cancer Diagnosis Grandmother's Death Built House/Moved Sister Divorce, Sister's Suicide Estrangement Teen Daughter Highschool, Boyfriend, College LA Job

REBOOT — New Home, New Job, Moved to Texas

FACING 50 — Doubt, Depression, Despair

MARATHON

DISCOVERY — Wayne Dyer, Redefined Dream!

Is that my whole life story? Not even close! But that was quite enough of a roller coaster ride wasn't it? And did you feel the ebb and flow? Yep, you guessed it. This is the lifebeat of love and fear. This is where you will re-learn that you have your own life's compass embedded in your soul.

Plotting your lifebeat will show you *when* you made the choice between love and fear. It will also help you understand why you are here and what you have come to learn.

Let's get started.

LIFEMAPPING EXPLORATION #2

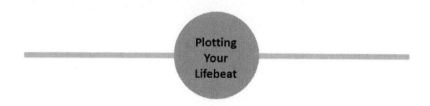

Centering Reminder: As in the last milestone exercise, the same guidelines apply:

1. Give yourself a time limit
2. Try not to overthink it
3. Try not to self-edit – write whatever comes
4. Don't worry about the chronology
5. Be gentle with yourself

OK, here are the steps:

1. **Identify:** Take a look at your milestones that you plotted out from our previous exercise. Re-imagine the "YOU" you were when that experience occurred.

Think about the year this event took place and what was going on in the world around you. Where were you when this happened? Were you a teenager or adult? Was this an action or decision you made for yourself or did someone or something do it for you?

2. **Evaluate:** As you consider these surrounding conditions, here's a key question to ask yourself: What was the result of each of those actions or decisions at that time... did they take you to a place of love or fear? Did you make the choice based on joyful expectations? Or did you do it to be safe, or appease the expectations of others? Did it take you to a place of happiness or sadness? Or did you make it in the effort to check a box or because you thought it was the safer choice?

3. **Plot:** You can create arcs for your Lifebeat that reflect the level of the fear or happiness that you felt, as this will also be an indicator of how impactful and important this particular event had on you. There are a number of ways to lay this out on paper for yourself, but following my example above will help you track your own illustration of your lifebeat. As you can see in my map, I had fairly consistent "happiness beats" on my path of love and connection. But on my fear milestones, there were big beats on my journey that really pushed me towards fear and disconnection.

When you are done, take inventory of how your map is coming to life, and ask yourself this:

What Is the Story Your Lifebeat Is Trying to Tell You?

Notes: Plotting out your life beat is not an exact science. The key is to step back and look at *why* that decision was made. What was your heart compass truly telling you? What were you feeling at that moment when you set your first foot in that college dorm, or took that walk down the aisle, took that job, or decided to get pregnant?

If you spend a little time on each one, you'll find that there is a relatively clear distinction of why you made a decision and how a particular event impacted your life.

Understanding the Love and Fear Scale:

As you work through plotting your lifebeat, it can also help to explore the "scale" of emotions that run between love and fear.

We have all heard about the "Law of Attraction." It is said, that it is the most powerful law of the universe, and governs all life forces. Einstein proved that everything in the universe is made up of energy (seen as well as unseen) and vibrates at a certain frequency. Humans also vibrate at a certain energy frequency, and your thoughts, feelings and beliefs determine the "vibration" of that energy. High vibrations like joy, appreciation and optimism sit on the LOVE spectrum of emotion. Lower energy vibrations sit on the FEAR spectrum and include emotions like hate, jealousy and sadness.

The more closely aligned your overall vibrational energy is to love, the better you feel. The closer you feel to fear, the lower your vibration and the worse you feel.

Here's one way to look at your "emotional scale" which runs from #1 Joy, Love and Empowerment to #22 Fear, Grief and Depression.

But we control the power of both the extent and impact of that emotion, and ultimately, the power it has to influence our experience. Let me explain what I mean...

The best explanation of how to understand and harness the law of attraction that I have ever encountered, is from the teachings of Abraham, a channeled group of non-physical beings brought forth by Esther Hicks. (Yeah, you just read that, but hang in there with me, I promise not to make this weird.) Since the early eighties, Esther and her late husband Jerry have shared the teachings of Abraham through their live events, recordings and many books. For me, their teachings have always sparked an inner "knowingness" that speaks to my soul.

According to Abraham, understanding our "emotional scale" or how we are feeling emotionally, is the best barometer to help shift our life experiences.

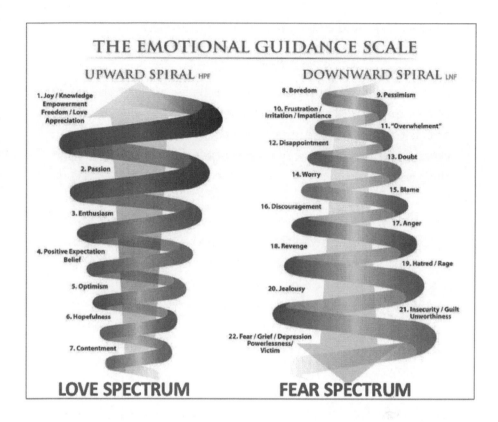

THE EMOTIONAL GUIDANCE SCALE

UPWARD SPIRAL HPF   DOWNWARD SPIRAL LNF

1. Joy / Knowledge Empowerment Freedom / Love Appreciation

8. Boredom

9. Pessimism

10. Frustration / Irritation / Impatience

11. "Overwhelment"

12. Disappointment

13. Doubt

2. Passion

14. Worry

15. Blame

3. Enthusiasm

16. Discouragement

17. Anger

4. Positive Expectation Belief

18. Revenge

19. Hatred / Rage

5. Optimism

20. Jealousy

21. Insecurity / Guilt Unworthiness

6. Hopefulness

22. Fear / Grief / Depression Powerlessness/ Victim

7. Contentment

LOVE SPECTRUM   **FEAR SPECTRUM**

This was also the first time that I learned about the very simple principles of understanding the impact of our relationship with love and fear. And that we can control our thoughts in a way that allows us to get, be and have more of what we want in our lives.

Focus on things that make us feel good, and more *good* comes in. Focus on things that don't feel good and we experience more things that don't feel good.

According to Abraham, if you think a thought for as little as 17 seconds, the law of attraction will bring another "like" thought to it. The longer you think a thought...the more thoughts within that energy will come to you. For example, if you wake up in the middle of the night and start thinking about a problem you are having, say your job, or a relationship, and you focus on it for as little as 17 seconds, more thoughts on the fear scale will also come to you.

And if you think a thought long enough, it becomes a belief. "A belief," Abraham says, "is just a thought you keep thinking." So, you have the power to change your beliefs, and thereby your point of attraction any time. You just need to figure out a way to change what you spend your time thinking.

This was such a huge lesson for me. It was then that I started to really watch my thoughts. I mean think about it. You have the power to decide for yourself at any point in time, what you think, and how you feel...about anything! It's like what Eleanor Roosevelt said about how "no one can make you feel inferior without your consent."

Remember always that you have the power to feel anything you want to feel. It is your choice and yours alone. Your power is in the present moment.

As we begin to dive in to understand our milestones, and the influence of love and fear on our experiences, it's important to know about the emotional scale of our emotions.

All of our emotions have different vibrational frequencies, and are indicators of your alignment with positive or negative energy. Your "emotional scale" is your GPS on where you are on the spectrum between love and fear. Considering the two extreme ends of this emotional scale, you could ask yourself, "Do I feel powerful, or do I feel powerless?"

When we are most aligned with who we are, meaning we are most connected with our soul, our source energy, the essence of who we are as souls, our emotions fall mostly on the left side of this spectrum. When we feel joy, optimism and helpful...we feel good...we are aligned with love and positivity. This creates an energetic "match" to other things in the positive energy field...that attracts other positive people, experiences and outcomes into our path. The better we feel...the more betterment is attracted into our experiences...and the more likely we are to "manifest" the things that will bring us more joy. Like attracts alike.

Here's what I love about understanding the "emotional scale." You can always choose a thought that feels better than the one you are currently feeling. For example, the feeling of anger can be a relief for someone who is in a state of grief. And frustration is one ring higher up on the scale than feeling overwhelmed.

From this perspective, the idea is no matter where you are emotionally, you should try to "reach for the thought or emotion that feels better." When you are aware you are feeling a strong negative emotion, try to identify the emotion. Sometimes, it's easier to start with the two extreme ends of the spectrum.

Ask yourself: Do I feel Fear or Appreciation? Belief or Disappointment? Once you have found your place on the emotional scale, your work is to try to find thoughts that give you a slight feeling of relief.

Finding the perfect word to describe how you feel is not important, but feeling through the emotion is the key to identifying where you are on the emotional scale. And finding ways to improve the feeling is even more important. We'll work more on that later in the book when we begin realigning our past experiences with positive affirmations that will shift the law of attraction in your favor.

For now, knowing about the scale of emotion offers you a powerful tool to help pinpoint the spectrum of emotions between love and fear, and as you look at each milestone, you can better pinpoint the source of your feelings and how these may influence the power of your attraction to a good or not so good experience. So many of us just don't know or pay attention to our own feelings (me included) and yet they are the very compass the helps us navigate our life's path...they are the GPS of our soul.

Understanding the Law of Attraction

Law of attraction is also a phrase linked to "manifestation," a seemingly "magical force" that can be summoned to help us get/be/achieve what we desire. For all the mystery that may surround this idea, it's a pretty simple concept. It's what my Mom always said. "What you focus on, grows." Focusing on your worries, perpetuates the fear, while focusing on gratitude allows your mind to expand and bring in more connection to love and the source of who you really are.

We all inwardly know this...so why do we get caught up in it? My feeling is that we just forget that the only time we can control is the present or the *now*. The only emotion we can control is in the now. Our power truly is in the now.

Let's try various emotions on and see how they feel, shall we?

Worry, doubt and fear are emotions about potential **future outcomes,** and reflect **low energy vibrations** on the FEAR SPECTRUM. Blame, Anger, Disappointment, reflect **judgements about past experience**s, and also live in the low end of the FEAR SPECTRUM.

These emotions feel dark and heavy, don't they? There's a weight to them. They make your heart hurt.

Hopefulness, Optimism and Positive Expectation are also emotions about potential *future* outcomes, but are **high energy vibrations** on the LOVE SPECTRUM. Appreciation and Enthusiasm are also **judgements about past experiences,** but they live on the high energy vibrations of the LOVE SPECTRUM.

The emotions feel light and bright...beckoning...alive. They offer a sweet invitation to visit tomorrow. They are sunny, alive and welcoming. They make your heart happy.

Again, as Abraham said, "a belief is just a thought you keep thinking." So how you think, is how you feel. And how you feel is what you attract.

The beauty of this is It's 100% within your control. At any point, no matter what is happening to or around us, we have the power to choose our reaction to it, and pick a different thought.

Think about it the next time someone triggers you by cutting you off on the highway or saying something that makes you feel inferior. You can choose to embrace the feeling of road rage, anger, blame, or self-doubt. Alternatively, you can reach for the thought that makes you feel better. Instead of thinking, "I hope that idiot hits a tree," you could simply say to yourself, "I'm having a great morning. I'm not going to let that situation bring me down. I'm going to let that person take his bad attitude elsewhere. I choose to be happy."

I'm not asking you to be Mother Theresa. I'm merely suggesting how you can take a nice little ride up the emotional scale from Revenge to Irritation, which will give you control of any situation you are in- every time. It's not easy to catch yourself...but when you do it gives you the feeling of sweet power over your own emotional destiny...because your only job, is to do your best to stay as close to love as possible.

I can tell you that it works, because it's the power that I used that morning in my bedroom when I couldn't get out of bed. I used it when I faced my divorce, my son's cancer diagnosis, my sister's suicide. I could not control the situation...but I could control the weight of how it ultimately impacted me emotionally. Which allowed me to have the strength I needed to take on the soul impacting role that was most important... to help others when possible.

Getting from a place of grief, powerlessness and unworthiness is the hardest work we will ever have to do for ourselves. And the only way to get there is through the tiny steps of reaching up and out of the darkness toward that light of love...which is always there. One reach at a time. One step at a time.

Here's an example of how understanding the emotional scale helped shift Ellen and Liz's understanding of their Lifemapping experiences.

ELLEN & LIZ'S STORY: Realigning Love

Ellen came to the workshop with her best friend Liz. It was early January and they had both made resolutions to do something that would help them better align their thinking for the year ahead.

Liz said she lived in outright fear of the law of attraction and blamed herself for manifesting the negative things in her life because she did not know how to "use the law correctly." She had recently gone through a series of radical changes, including a divorce, loss of a job and some health issues.

Liz had also escaped an abusive family situation when she was young, by enlisting in the army when she was 18. And while she initially hated the regimented life on the military base, she got to see the world, and ultimately used the training to secure a job she loved.

When Ellen went through the Lifemapping exercise, she had a hard time discerning some of her life experiences as definitively fitting into the bucket of love or fear. She gave the example of her first marriage beginning as a reach toward love and a new life with her new husband. But over time, it led to infidelity and divorce.

In both cases, Liz and Ellen initially "reached" for their life milestones with the intention of moving toward a "better" experience, but the key is to look at the emotion at the *origin* of the reach. *What prompted the decision for each of these experiences?* Did they really come from a place of happiness aligned with the heart, or was the choice made to escape an unhappy or uncomfortable situation? This is why we call this a heartbeat...because the heart always knows and hears its quiet knowing.

This is where it gets interesting.

For Ellen, when she really stepped back and remembered making her decision to get married, she understood that, while she thought she went into her engagement from a place of love, when she really tapped into her heart, she realized that the decision to walk down the aisle came from a place of her own insecurity. When she stepped back and accessed what was in her heart, she recognized she had been (and still was) deeply shy, and had never had a boyfriend. With a renewed understanding of her younger self's fear of abandonment, she understood that, when the opportunity came, she took it, fearing no one else might come along again to ask her. So, while this marriage milestone might have initially appeared to have been one that was reaching toward love, at its core, the decision came from a place of fear.

This was a huge revelation for Ellen...because it helped her understand why her marriage was ultimately unhappy and unfulfilling for her. She had reached towards that relationship from a place of self-doubt and fear of abandonment.

So, what had outwardly appeared as a LOVE milestone, was actually a FEAR milestone for her.

Liz, on the other hand, knew that her "escape" to the military was to leave behind a dysfunctional family and that she enlisted to get out of a fearful situation.

Liz reached out to life in the military from a place of courage. She knew that she needed to take a bold step to leave her terrible childhood behind her, so she made the hard decision to enlist in the military. Enlisting was a choice toward self-betterment; it was a huge move that showed that she loved herself enough to make an uneasy choice in the hopes of a positive outcome. Therefore, it was a LOVE MILESTONE. The key to her milestone is that she was reaching toward her own self-empowerment.

She went from a place of shame and anger to a place of courage by firmly and unequivocally saying "no" to the awful situation in her home and reaching for a better life. And though it was challenging, this led Liz forward to a more enriching life path that was aligned with her soul's purpose.

All of this said, it is so important to remember that these choices DO NOT make us right or wrong because, as we will discover in the next chapter, this is our life school. Since we have chosen these experiences and enlisted the help of our soul squad before coming into these lifetimes, we must fully immerse ourselves in the school of life. We want to participate in both the joy and the painful moments to give us opportunities to choose and to learn. We are all here as souls wanting to grow and evolve.

PLAYING OUT YOUR MOVIE: Lifebeat Recap:

OK, now it's time to play out what you've learned so far through this Lifebeat experience in an activity I call "The movie of your mind."

Take a moment to sit restfully and do the "life review" of your milestones. See the child you were, that evolved into the teen, the young adult, to adult...all the key moments that stand out for you as your life unfolded to where you are today.

And as you do this, imagine you are sitting in a movie theater and you are not in fact yourself, your body, or your own experience. Instead, you are just seated in the audience, observing someone else's story, unfolding on the movie screen.

As you playback your "life's movie," consider the following:

1. How do you feel about the main character of the story? How would you describe their story?
2. Are there key protagonists and antagonists who have been part of their story?
3. Are there challenges that they are consistently dealing with? Is there a common thread throughout? Can you identify a lesson they are presented with over and over again?
4. What are the highlights/best moments in the story?
5. What were the lowest points in the story?
6. Where would you like to see the story go from here?
7. How would you write the best possible ending to their movie?

Take Some Notes. How Does This Make You Feel About the "Movie Star" (You)?

As you reflect on this part of your LifeMap experience, reward yourself for your willingness to go this far and take this important assessment of the role that love and fear play in your life. Embrace the power that is your ability to choose everything that happens to you from the vantage point of the emotional scale.

You ARE the creator of your own experience.

Take a moment and acknowledge your strength. Thank your heart and your soul for the bravery that you have exemplified by taking this journey.

You are, in every sense, a life warrior, just for showing up... for making the effort...for being willing to wake up every day and begin again.

To conclude this very important work, I offer you this loving Soulfirmation:

 SOULFIRMATION #3

"I hold within myself an inner compass
that always clearly guides my path and shows me my direction towards love or fear.
It holds all of the clarity and guidance I need along my journey
to walk boldly and make decisions
always in the interest of my higher good.
Each milestone I create along my path gives me the opportunity to learn and fulfill my purpose —
what I have come to do, and what I have come to learn."

Your heart is hugging you now, can you feel it?
(I am too.)
Namaste, my friend. Let's keep going!

SOUL GOODY BAG

Here are some resources mentioned in this chapter for you for further exploration:

Ask and it is Given: Learning to Manifest Your Desires. Ester and Jerry Hicks (The Teachings of Abraham) 2004, which presents the teachings of the nonphysical entity Abraham, will help you learn how to manifest your desires to live the joyous and fulfilling life you deserve.

As you read, you'll come to understand how your relationships, health issues, finances, career concerns, and more are influenced by the Universal laws that govern your time-space-reality—and you'll discover powerful processes that will help you go with the positive flow of life.

It's your birthright to live a life filled with everything that is *good*—and this book will show you how to make it so in every way!

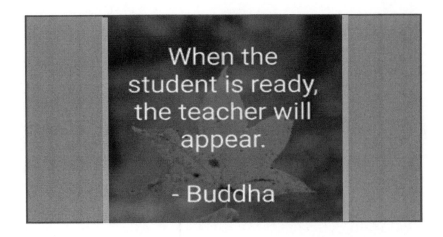

When the student is ready, the teacher will appear.

- Buddha

CHAPTER 4

IDENTIFYING YOUR SOUL SQUAD

When I took a step back to look at my milestones and my lifebeat, it became clear that I wasn't on this journey by myself. Through almost every experience and life event, there were clearly people who had an impact and assisted in molding my beliefs, feelings, ideas and perspectives. They helped shape the vision I had of the world, and the vision I had of myself.

Every person who comes into our lives has the opportunity to teach us something and impact our life's path. From the coffee barista who serves up your latte with a smile every morning, to that two-timing boyfriend who broke your heart, to the high school music teacher who helped you find your singing voice, to the boss who severely overworked you and taught you how to create personal boundaries, we all have special teachers who come into our lives at specific times to help us make decisions between love and fear.

To our conscious mind, these may seem like people who really came into our experiences arbitrarily, by fate, accident or happenstance. But ah, if you could only see behind the curtain of the universe, you would identify these souls as carefully chosen members of your soul tribe, all choreographed with perfectly orchestrated roles and synchronicity by your own divine choosing.

Gosh, how I love that last sentence! Let me convince you that it's true.

We're all afflicted with earthbound amnesia that has us forget the intention from which we came, that is, until life's encounters with our soul squad offer us a chance to wake up.

Sound odd, far-fetched, a little too "out there"? The language may sound a little lofty, but I assure you, this is really the way it goes. If you can open up the aperture on the lens of your life just a little more, you'll discover a beautifully deep, multi-dimensional universe that is far richer and more meaningful than could ever meet your human eye.

Let's dig into this fascinating world of soul synchronicity, shall we?

This chapter will weave together your key milestones with the people and influencers in your life and help you define the roles they have played in your lifetime, so far.

Together, we will do the following:

1. Define the Purpose and Role of Your Soul Squad
2. Learn how to recognize both the physical and non-physical members of your Soul Squad
3. Identify which Soul Squad members most influenced you and Line them up with your milestones

4. Learn how to ask your angels and guides for guidance

Our soul squad offers points of light in our carefully woven tapestry of experience as we make our way down life's path. This helps us choose and chisel the evolving facets of our being such as what we believe about ourselves. This chapter will help weave together your key milestones with the key people and influencers in your life (big and small). It will also help to identify the roles these key people have played in your life so far. You'll discover how your soul pod and the people you attract into your life are huge reflections of who are you are as a soul. You will also gain insight into how these individuals function as mirrors which reflect your life's purpose.

Why We Choose a Soul Squad:

As I shared in Chapter two, I believe that we all come into our "earth school" and have chosen our teachers, classmates, and the "lessons" we want to study. Our soul squad is specifically chosen to play "a part" in our lifetime, with mutual intentions to share experiences with us. These shared experiences provide opportunities to learn and grow from each other.

Some of these souls will come in and play a role through the majority of our entire lifespan, while others may come and go for certain periods of time or at designated points along the way. They could be your child, your birth mother, your yoga teacher or your boss. Regardless of their chosen role, each of these people have come to share relevant moments along our life's path to help shape our feelings about ourself, other humans, and the world.

Finding Your Squad

Your soul squad can also be your "soul team." Meaning that you may often reincarnate with the same group of people throughout many different lifetimes. This is because you have made a spiritual choice to be connected on a "soul level" because of a deep and eternal love that you have for each other. In each life experience you take on a specific role, sharing life lessons through different personalities and experiences. This can even mean reversing roles from one lifetime to another.

Your Mother, for example, may have been your child in a previous life, and perhaps struggled with unresolved issues of communication or a lack of understanding. When you completed that lifetime and did your life review, the two of you may have agreed to come back with exchanged roles, in order to better understand how to relate to each other in this lifetime and work through and resolve those differences, so not to carry them into the next life.

Oftentimes, we are reunited with fellow souls in multiple lifetimes because we just work really well together. For example, a soul squad might continue to stay with each other through many lifetimes because they know that there is great connective love between them. This love will be a reminder on a soul level that will best help them learn in each lifetime.

But like any good "sequel" the idea is to switch up the plot each time, to keep the experiences and learnings deep and enriching...all with the intention of completing lessons during our earth school days to graduate and "move up a learning level" after each lifetime.

Getting the Band Back Together

So, before we are born, we create the "master plan" with our squad. We get our gang together to decide what each life "plot" will be about. What are the main lessons we want to learn? What is the best role I can play within the group to lovingly assist the development and expansion of each soul? And how do I plan the best opportunities and circumstances for me to grow and become a more enlightened and loving soul?

And yes, we choose to experience drama. Pain, suffering, loss and sadness are lessons we choose (yes choose) because they offer us the opportunity to learn the biggest lessons.

Wait ... what? Hold on there for just one crazy second, life mapper lady... did you say people actually CHOOSE their pain and suffering? Do you mean it's planned?

In one word, YEP, but not totally.

The idea is that while we do actually create a plan for our lives with our angels, guides and soul squad with clear intentions of what we want to do, be and experience, we always have free will to make whatever choices we want when we actually get here. Hint: It all has to do with the choice between fear and love.

Free will is always our extra roll of the dice. It is our "plan B," where we can change our mind, or just sit the decision out altogether. But each time we do that...we feel the groove. And I promise you, we always inwardly know if love or fear was the judge of our jury.

Creating Your Life's Blueprint

There is no better book for understanding how we plan our life experiences, than "Your Soul's Plan" by Robert Schwartz.

For me, it was the most life-changing book I've ever read to help understand the meaning of our life's purpose.

Robert approaches his work differently than that of a past life regressionist. Instead of taking people back to review their prior past life experiences, he takes people back to revisit the space BETWEEN lives...right before they are born. This is the time where he believes we have in-depth conversations with our spirit guides and the other souls that we will share our lives with. This is the place and time we design the blueprint of our soul.

"The planning we do before birth is far reaching and detailed," Rob writes. "It includes but goes well beyond the selection of life challenges. We choose our parents (and they choose us), when and where we will incarnate, the schools we will attend, the people we will meet, the relationships we will have. If you have ever felt you already know someone you just met, it may well be true. That person was probably part of your pre-birth planning."

Robert also explains the reason why we sometimes get the feeling of déjà vu, as an example of us remembering tiny morsels of our pre-planned experiences that we've predestined and pre-seen before we were born.

Through the thousands of regressions, he has done, Robert found a similar theme was recounted each and every time. "Everyone has a divine purpose, a reason for being here, that includes but goes well beyond our own learning. That is, we plan life challenges not only to remember who we really are, but also to share ourselves, our unique essence, with one another."

The idea that we may plan our life experiences ahead of time, or at least the opportunities to learn the lessons we need to learn for our soul's growth, transformed the way I looked at life. If I had planned to face the pain of my divorce, my son's cancer journey, my sister's suicide…was there a greater, more divine and purposeful reason for it happening?

Could it be a quest to learn forgiveness? To face my gravest fear and carry my child from disease to wellness? To use my grief and loss as a tool to heal my spirit and share what I've learned with others? Could I have selected all of it as my earthly test to expand my ability to love unconditionally?

For me, this recognition of this undeniable truth still brings tears to my eyes. It has taken me to a place of profound gratitude for every battle, and seemingly horrific life event that has happened to me. None of it has been random events of unfortunate luck or bad choices. It is all a result of my courageous soul signing up for a life filled with opportunities to share the loving, brave, powerful light that is me. With the profound recognition of this soul truth, I send love to my ex-husband, and to my son's cancer diagnosis and my angel sister, for their beautiful, loving co-creation in my life, knowing I signed up for it all.

And I am so very, very grateful.

And that, is why I am so honored to have you here with me on this life-mapping journey, so you too can discover your soul's blueprint as well.

As Robert shared, there are so many lessons that we have come here to learn and to teach. Tolerance, healing, truthful communication, compassion, faith, and resilience are just a few of them. "Each soul comes here to be the love they are. Courageous souls, one and all," is how Robert concludes his final chapter. So well said.

Read the book. Trust me, it will change your life, and your vision of your life's purpose, forever. Amen.

Let me share the story of a very special Soul Seeker named Lisa and how her heavenly Momma and earthly Aunt became her soul tribe on the other side and the role they played in opening her heart to her life's purpose.

Lisa's Seeker Story: Signs from Our Soul Mommas

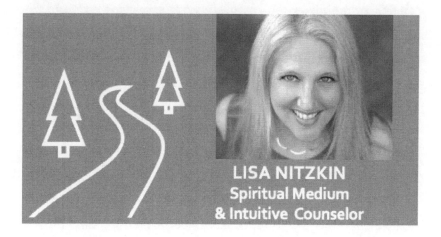

LISA NITZKIN
Spiritual Medium
& Intuitive Counselor

"My Mom died of cancer when I was seven years old. At the time, I was too young to understand what death really was, and I felt scared and lost for a long time. Gratefully, I was guided by my spiritual Aunt who helped me understand that my mom was still with me even without her physical presence.

The day after my Mother passed, there was a rainbow in the sky. My Aunt reassured me that it was a sign that my Mom was smiling with me. From that day on, I carried that symbol as a message of love from her and since then, the rainbow has appeared at every single celebration or time that I needed it.

The rainbow has also appeared when I've had hard decisions to make or when I've been in need of her guidance. It never fails. She even shows up with my rainbows during non-rainbow seasons just to let me know she is still with me. It has provided much comfort as I know that she has never really left my side.

As I grew older, that feeling of "knowing" and see-ing a variety of signs became stronger and I found myself having psychic experiences that just couldn't be explained. I knew my mom's presence was real and that I had connected to my intuitive abilities and she was helping me navigate through this newfound under-standing of my soul's truth.

I began to use that "knowing" by tapping into all of my energy senses and listening to my inner guidance. I was hearing and seeing messages that became clearer as I practiced. I started reading for others and found that many validating messages were helping people heal through their personal losses by connecting into the energy of their deceased loved ones. It became my life's purpose to help people understand that there is no true separation between this life and the afterlife and that we are never alone."

In Lisa's case, it was her Mother and her Aunt who took on the important soul squad roles that helped inspire Lisa's path as a medium and healer. The tragic experience of losing her mother as a seven-year-old, was the catalyst for looking for the signs from the other side that ultimately taught her how to use her psychic senses in order to follow the symbols of rainbows and better tune into the frequencies to be able to experience the messages and connections she so needed from her mom.

With her Aunt's help, Lisa learned to seek out those signs, and fine tune her gifts to share messages with people from their loved ones on the other side to help them heal as well. This is an inspiring example of how our soul squad helps support us through experiences to expand our own growth so we can help others.

Your Soul Squad Is Both Physical and Non-Physical

In addition to those who have taken up the charge to be with us in our physical lifetime, there are also those who have signed up to be our non-physical teachers and protectors. Part of our soul's plan before we came into our earthly bodies, was defining who would be with us on the earthly playing field, as well as those who would be watching and cheering from your heavenly grandstand.

Simply put: We have got quite a mix of souls in our squad – who have signed up to play their parts from both the physical and non-physical realms.

Angels and Spirit Guides:

Before we take this little joyride to find your soul tribe, try, if you can, to place any preconceived feelings about spiritual religion in the back seat for just a moment. I know this can be a tricky subject, especially if you grew up going to a church that loomed high with those willowy flyers hovering with huge wings and halos in and around the religious statues and stained-glass windows.

It's a shame, in a way, that these ethereal protectors are mostly portrayed as spiritual deities, valiantly fighting off serpents trying to steal away human souls ... or bemoaning the imminent death of a saint being tormented, or serving as a messenger delivering a heavenly proclamation or assignment (probably also leading to death and suffering). I was slightly terrified of my bedtime prayers fearing that calling upon them would mean I'd be whisked away before the lights went out.

But it's such a better story than we've been taught.

Your "Heavenly" Task Force

In addition to your earthly soul tribe, before you begin your new human lifetime, you also line up your celestial tag-team. This is your crew that will be your wingmen (and wing women) on the other side - your entourage of angels and guides who'll keep their eye on the "big picture" of your life. These are your "invisible friends" who are just as real as your earthly team, and are there to guide, guard and light your way as you navigate your earthly journey.

So, what is the difference between angels and guides? I believe that we are all given both. And there are about as many different beliefs about the different kinds of angels and guides, as there are...well, angels and guides.

Here's My Take:

1. Spirit guides

Your spirit guides are extremely close companions who play a very special role in your life's journey. These are **souls who have once lived on earth** who understand the human experience and can closely relate to our joys and challenges. Think of them as "spiritual specialists" or your "celestial concierge" who are assigned to you to help navigate all of the challenges and lessons you have signed up for in your earth school. These Spirit Guides come and go as advisors as you need them. Some call spirit guides the little voice in our heads that can amplify our intuition as we make key decisions and life choices. They are the experts we can call on to guide us to the information we need in our decisions, for our healing, parenting, careers or relationships. They are there to help you attain your highest potential in your soul's evolution.

A spirit guide can be a soul you've had past life experiences with, who choose to remain in the spirit plane to be your guide from the non-physical. They might also be part of your earthly soul squad, who takes on the role of spirit guide after they pass on...like a grandparent or close friend, who remains connected to us to offer their continued guidance from the other side.

As we saw from her story, Lisa believes that her mom is one of her spirit guides. Their pre-life pact to form a deep bond on their earthly walk as mother and daughter, was the catalyst for Lisa's desire to seek signs of her mother's continued presence in her life. Ultimately this led to her work as a healer, medium and teacher who is helping thousands work through their grief and inspire their own beliefs on life after death.

2. Guardian angels

Their name implies who and what they are...messengers and protectors of light. Guardian angels are spirits who have been specifically assigned to watch over you for your entire lifetime. The biggest difference between guardian angels and spirit guides is that guardian angels **have never lived as human beings**. Instead, they've always existed in spirit. Therefore, they exist on a much higher energetic level than spirit guides.

These energetic beings are also assigned to you at birth, and many teachers believe that you have at least two guardian angels. While spirit guides assist you as expert teachers, guardian angels take on a more protective role. They are the light that watches over you and are with you in moments of danger or fear. The arch-angels, such as Raphael and Michael, live on the highest realms of the angel hierarchy, and can be called upon for healing and strength. Your guardian angel is the gatekeeper at your life's entrance and exit points. They lovingly watch over you as you make the precarious transition from heaven to earth, stay with you throughout every moment of your earthly pilgrimage, and are there to softly shepherd you through your transition back "home" again.

According to Alma Daniels, one of the co-writers of "Ask Your Angels: A Practical Guide to Working with the Messengers of Heaven to Empower and Enrich Your Life," there is no set way to connect with your angels. It doesn't have to be through prayer or meditation. You don't have to be seated in a church or holy ground. Rather, "they come to us very much on their own terms, appearing to us in ways that are very personal to each individual." (Ask Your Angels, p.5).

"Contact and conversation with your Angel," Alma writes, "is filled with all the tenderness and love and wonderment of discovering a best friend – known forever, but not seen in years. Talking with angels is an entirely natural relationship, although over the centuries it's become obscured by the belief that if you can't see something or touch it – it isn't real.

Now, at a time when we need help more than ever before, the angels are stepping forward once again. Interestingly, they tell us that it is because of reorganizations within their own domain that they are receiving instructions to make closer contact with us. Just as we are preparing ourselves for the enormous changes ahead, so the angels tell us that they are also evolving. As above, so below.

Their closer presence is deeply encouraging – just the helping hand for which so many of us have been praying. *The angels are here*. They are with us whether we believe in them or not. The universe works on a need-to-know basis; when we ask, we are answered. In talking to our angels, we extend and expand our capacity for growth and transformation – and we move closer to our destiny." (Ask You Angels p.5).

How exciting to know that our angels are just an "ask" away. And that they aren't just a symbol or part of a prayer that we learn as children. Calling upon our angels on our life's journey is and should continue to be part of an arsenal of spiritual allies that we call upon every day. Try it today, and see what signs and surprises show up for you.

3. Your "higher self"

One other celestial being that should not be overlooked is your very own dear, pure and powerful soul. This is the eternal, everlasting, ever-perfect you. The essence of your being that has always been and forever will be...Your Higher Self.

When we make our decision to incarnate into human form, we put on the robe of a physical body - this so called "birthday suit," with which we use as a "vehicle" to move around and experience the earth, is but a physical sheath with which cloaks our true selves, our true light, our true essence, and our infinite, authentic, higher selves.

This is the part of us that is our inner compass...that remembers why we came. It is the home of our aspiration, and inspiration, where our knowingness and our dreams live. We only need to go inside and listen quietly, casting aside our ego and our fears. That's where love and our infinite power resides. Deepak Chopra, the great author and expert in mind body healing once wrote "the higher self is whispering to you softly in the silence between your thoughts."

Spirit 911

Now that we understand this divine orchestration, how can we ever consider ourselves alone? We have so much help around us that we can call upon any time, for virtually anything we need.

Your spirit squad has been hand-picked and orchestrated by you and for you, and always has your back, both physically and virtually. Your higher self, your angels, your spirit guides is your life team of divine intelligence…. all with mutually chosen roles in helping you see, understand and fulfil your life's purpose. They are the multifaceted, multi-loving, multi-knowing part of ourselves that will always be there at our side and on the other side, guiding us with their gentle love and cheering us on.

At the end of this chapter, I'll show you how you can connect with your Spirit Guides and angels, and how to recognize the signs that they are sending your way.

But for now, let's get back down to earth.

Our Earthy Soul Squad

Our Soul Squad also includes members of our earth family. And as I've already mentioned, this is not limited to your physical family of parents, relatives and siblings. Your Soul squad also includes, friends, enemies, lovers and acquaintances. They can be those you've known for long periods of time as well as those who may only cross your path for an instant.

So how do we identify these special members who have decided to jump on the tribal tour bus?

Let's start with our earth family.

Whether or not you get along with your mom, sister, cousins or in-laws, trust me, chances are you all have come in with some very specific intentions for what you all want to learn from each other. As you look at your milestones, you will see that your family members have all had specific roles in teaching you lessons of love and fear. But it might also surprise you to know that you've all mutually selected to incarnate together in this lifetime, as well as previous ones.

Whether you get along or not, is, well... exactly the point. And the intensity of these feelings of love (affinity/admiration) and fear (dislike/anger) is a clue to the importance of the soul contract you have with them.

Take my family for example. I have no doubt that this is definitely not my first incarnation rodeo with my mother and grandmother. They clearly came to expand their ancient wisdom in this lifetime and water the roots of our familial spiritual learning as well as fulfill their own roles in moving our collective consciousness and enlightenment forward. I'm also certain that my extremely wise daughter Lauren has been an ongoing member of my spiritual squad through many lifetimes. She has been my coach and counselor, and has such a calm, soothing presence over me. If I am seeking solid and practical advice, she is the first person I turn to. She too, is an emerging spiritual seeker, but with far more of a laser beam focus on who she is than I've ever had.

While her father and I divorced when she was just a baby and it was a very difficult parting of ways for us, I have been able to readjust my blame and ultimately come to a place of gratitude for his role in my soul squad. Afterall, he helped me co-create Lauren's existence in the world. I recognize that much of her patience and grounded-ness has come from being the daughter of divorced parents. Having this understanding has also helped me release some of the guilt that I carried with me after the divorce, because I know we both chose this experience together.

As you begin to map your experiences, you too will see that the significance of these people and the interactions you share will be the clues that will help you identify your own personal soul squad.

Recognizing People in Your Soul Tribe

I have found, "rule of thumb" is that there are some absolutely outstanding clues for recognizing our soul mates. And I'll also warn you that you might not like some of them! But I offer them here, because as your soul map begins to come alive with your true life's story, and you begin to identify your soul squad, the lines between your so-called friends and enemies will begin to blur. You'll start to see the true role of those who brought fear, heartache and pain into your life were just as important soul mates as those who brought you love, joy and gosh-how-did-I-ever-live-without-them-happiness.

Here Are a Few to Try on for Size:

1. **The Teachers: They have taught you a specific life lesson about love or fear.** These are the members of your soul squad who'll probably come to mind first. They are the ones that "see you" differently. On the love side, these may be your parents, your spouse, or a best friend. On the fear side, it might be the bully that targeted you in school, the boss that

fired you, the ex who told you that you were too fat to love. Teachers are the people that caused you to define how you feel about yourself, and reinforced your connectedness or disconnectedness to your soul's purpose.

In addition to your "teachers," there are also another part of your squad that I like to call your "Soul Influencers." While they may not immediately have come to mind while plotting out our milestones, they play a formative role in formulating how we feel about the world and hold up a mirror to ourselves. Here are a few examples.

2. **The Triggers: You dislike them almost immediately**. They seem to have been placed in your path as permanent pebbles in your shoe. Could be that girl with the perfect body in your yoga class, or that condescending, ego-tist college professor. Your mother-in-law perhaps? You know who they are. They push your buttons. They are sandpaper. They poke your ugly. They are the contrastors...the ones that seemingly contradict your "rightness" and "beliefs." Ah but they have a role to play...bless them one and all. They are there as mirrors of your own beliefs, to show the opposite view. What do they trigger in you? Whatever it is, there's an opportunity there to shine a light of love.

3. **The Kindreds:** These are the oppositive of the triggers. You are attracted to them almost immediately. You feel as if you've known them forever. They turn on a light inside you. There is happiness and goodness in their company. You feel like you've known them

forever. "You're my peep," you think, as you sit down with this new-found friend over coffee. There is an instant feeling of knowingness, connection, warmth and familiarity. And it lingers and lasts. It's like boom... you're kin! They are there as mirrors of the love that is already there within you. With them, your inner love light shines even brighter.

4. **The Disrupters:** They are those ones who come in and out of your life at unexpected times and places to shake things up – the doctor that provides a lifechanging diagnosis, the person who rear-ends your car and sues you. The brother or sister you didn't know you had. The unexpected pregnancy. These are the souls who turn your life unexpectedly upside down...that bring in the "wait, what?" Whether they bring happiness or heartburn and ebb in and out like the tide, there's lessons there, gift wrapped for you...and it's almost always a mirror. These disruptors will often expose the fear that lives inside of you and provide an opportunity for you to turn that fear into growth.

5. **The Connectors:** They introduce you to someone, something or an idea that makes a huge impact: the friend of a friend that puts you in touch with that perfect job opportunity, the hairdresser that sets you up on the blind date. The person on the airplane that shares a book, story or experience that shifts everything. These are the souls who come along to serve as the catalyst for change... for making a decision that can set you down a whole new life path.

As you begin thinking about who these very special soul mates are in your life, softly open your heart to the possibility that you had a life pre-birth planning session with them, and that the love or fear opportunities each of them brought to you were ones that you agreed to as a team ahead of time.

If your heart can accept this as a possibility, can this change how you look at them? Does it reframe the role of joy or sorrow they brought to your life? How would your perspective of this milestone and soul "mate" change your current belief about them?

Therein, lies the golden threads you are weaving in the tapestry of your life.

Lifemapper Stories: Todd's Story and the Soul Mate Who Made the Forever Impact

TODD'S STORY: The Soul Mate that Made Forever Impact

Todd had grown up in a tiny mid-western suburb just south of Kansas City. He was the sixth child and final offspring in his family and was struggling to find a way to stand out in a long line of his older, successful siblings. He recalled his memories of his young adult life with inner sadness. "By the time I came along, my parents were tired of raising kids. They were both working hard to support us, so we were pretty much on our own. My older sister was our drill sergeant. She kept us in line at home, made sure we did our homework and didn't straggle too far off."

All of Todd's brothers and sisters were high achievers. They did well in school, excelled in sports, and had lots of friends. Todd tried following in their footsteps, but just couldn't keep up. "I felt like a drifter...like I was an afterthought that didn't matter much."

Todd recognized his siblings and parents as influencers in his early life, but not as his soul squad. As he looked back on those formative years as a young man, searching for members of his true soul family, his eyes teared up when he remembered Margie.

"I look back on my life now and can truly trace the people who made all the difference for me with their tiny acts of kindness. Things that seemed so small at the time that literally transformed my life experience and the path I chose. Margie was that soul guide for me."

Todd told the story of how he was sitting alone in the high school cafeteria when Margie, the cafeteria lady, was cleaning up. "Why aren't you in class?" she asked with a warm smile. "I come and sit here instead of study hall." Todd answered. "It smells good in here."

Margie laughed. "Well, that's a first," she said. "Most people don't appreciate the smell of cafeteria kitchen food. But I try to bring my own little style to it. You are smelling my own special spaghetti sauce. I add my little spice of life to every dish I make."

"When she said that, her 'spice of life,'" Todd said, "Her whole face lit up. It was like a secret only she knew. Now I see it as her own inner spark as she talked about what she loved to do."

Margie liked to ask questions. "Do you like food?" "I guess," Todd answered. "Ah, that's not an answer," she said. "Let's try an experiment." She went into the school kitchen and came back with a small ceramic bowl and a wooden spoon. "Try this."

The taste was transformational. Todd could see the spices, the aroma of the tangy warm tomatoes. The swirl of the slightest hint of parmesan cheese. This wasn't food. It was an experience. "Wow." he said.

"This is my recipe," Marg said was unhidden pride. "It is the thing I do. The gift I was born to offer to everyone. It won't make me a million dollars, but it makes people feel good. And that's what it really means to feel blessed." He never ever forgot the way she said it.

"How do you make this?" he asked.

"Ahhh," Margie said with satisfaction. "Now that's an answer."

From that day on, with the school's permission, he spent my study hall in the cafeteria kitchen, learning how to cook with Margie. We started with the spaghetti sauce, and moved on to macaroni and cheese, lentil soup, salt butter biscuits, and pumpkin pie.

He would come home from school smelling like food and make the recipes for his family. "They finally saw me... and I **became me**. I found my calling...and haven't stopped cooking since."

Todd now owns several successful restaurants which also offer classes for aspiring chefs. He finished the exercise reflecting on how his role as a student in Margie's cooking class was a mutual soul exchange.

"I found out later that Margie had a son who had been a Marine and was killed overseas. He was only nineteen. I think I helped fill that void for her and gave her someone she could pass down her recipes to that would help continue her legacy of cooking.

While Todd spent only a few months in Margie's kitchen, the "spice of life" lesson stayed with him and helped him recognize the pact they made to inspire and support each other. Truly they were both soul mates who were able to heal and inspire each other to find a mutual path for their life's purpose.

Time to ID Your Squad:

Now that you've gotten the low down on all of the types of peeps in your soul squad and the potential role they can play in your lifetime, it's time to take your own personal inventory.

Here's a tip: Your soul squad is typically hovering around your biggest life milestones.

Let's go through some of mine on the next page as an example.

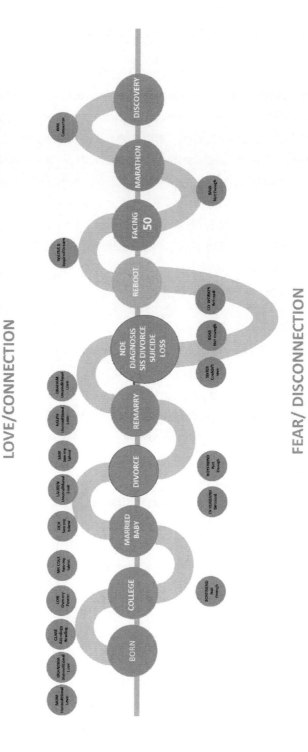

Looking back again at my big milestones, my squad was easy to spot.

My mother, my grandmother...who were my earthly Yoda's, my formative earth guides who, from the very beginning, nourished and nurtured me with inspirational, aspirational insights, ideas and ideology.

Then, the friends and teachers who entered during my literal earth school...my high school English teacher, Mr. Cole, who helped me find my creative voice. My best friend Lori who dared me to push my limits and test my wings.

All of those beginning experiences shined a light of love on my path.

Then, tougher lessons begin. With Bobby came my first heartbreak. The seeming "lack" of love presents itself and my lifebeat dips towards fear. My college escape is overwhelming, lonely and unfulfilling. I meet Jim. Reaching again back towards love, we marry. I subsequently get a new job and mentor, and my beautiful baby brings me back to hope and light.

Then betrayal throws me back into fear, retracking my thoughts and beliefs about my own worthiness. My identity is recast from coupled to single. I'm relabeled as "divorcee," and "single mother." Lifebeat dips again.

Can you see how my soul squad has influenced each milestone and lifebeat? And how each of them always offered me the opportunity with a choice of what to believe: fear or love.

So now you're ready to ID your squad.

Setting Your Intention

This is a powerful time to bless and give thanks to all the wonderful souls in your life who've contributed to your soul's progress so far. Whether they are playing a leading role in your life's "movie" or just an "extra," each has made a pre-life contract with you to be part of this experience.

Before you take this next important step on our life mapping journey, take a moment to center your thoughts with this soulfirmation:

 SOULFIRMATION #4

"I recognize all the people who come into my life are teachers.
I know everyone has offered me the gift of growth
And we are intertwined
by a mutual invitation to distinguish
between fear and love.
I am grateful for this opportunity to co-create these experiences
And remember why we are here in this lifetime together
as souls in search of our truest selves."

And exhale …. let us begin.

LIFEMAPPING EXPLORATION #3:

Identifying
Your
Soul Squad

> **Lifemapping Reminder:** As in the last milestone exercise, the same guidelines apply:
>
> 1. Give yourself a time limit – 20 minutes is a good goal.
> 2. As in our prior exercises, find a comfortable location and utilize materials that are fun and easy for you to work with.
> 3. Try not to overthink it or self-edit.
> 4. Don't worry about the chronology or timeline of events.
> 5. Be gentle with yourself – if this becomes too emotional for one sitting, you can divide this exercise into parts, or come back when you are ready.

OK – here we go! This is a four-step process:

1. **Identify:** Go back and take a look at your Key Milestones. Who were the people who were part of those events? Write down the names of the people you associate with those events.

2. **Evaluate:** What role did they play in your life? Even though you may now understand the "lessons" that they might have taught you now, think about the role that they played in your life at the time. How did they make you feel…. Love or Fear?

3. **Plot:** Place their name "above the line" if they invoke a feeling of Love/Connection or "below the line" if they connect with the feeling of Fear/Disconnection.

4. **Reflect:** This is the place where you can jot some quick notes in your journal about your soul squad.
   a. What other emotions come to mind when you think about that person?
   b. Were they a Teacher, Trigger, Kindred, Disrupter, Connector or Influencer?
   c. Was there a recurrence/repeat/pattern of the same kinds of people continually trying to teach you the same lessons over and over again?

d. What was the lesson they might have been trying to teach you? Have you learned it yet?

Take a few minutes to add any additional thoughts, reflections or insights to your journal. You may want to take a break now and let those thoughts and "aha's" digest. There is much to learn...and still so much to uncover. For now, revel in the landscape of your beautiful life portrait knowing that you are forever and, in this moment, surrounded by the unending love of your squad, guides, angels and soul mates. Through all of it, they are always at the center of your universe!

Lifemapper Stories: How Your Squad Influences Your Life's Path

NANCY'S STORY: Painting the Future on a New Canvas

Nancy's life began in a tiny suburb of Boston. She was an only child who lived in an affluent home. Her father was a well-known doctor, whose father was also a doctor before him, and their family lineage could be traced back to the Mayflower. He was ever-agitated and could only be seen in the late evenings, sitting in his study with his brandy and his newspaper. "He was the kind of man you didn't want to interrupt or even notice you were there." Nancy said. As she spoke, I could see the fear, ever-present, as if she were still there in the room with him.

Nancy explained that her mother was a frail, sickly woman who battled with anxiety and depression. "She also rarely spoke and sat most of the time in silence with her novels and her needlepoint." Nancy said. She remembered the loneliness throughout most of her childhood, with her only ally being her grandmother, who would take her to the theatre, art galleries and museums in the city.

For Nancy, these excursions were both magical and a relief- a full escape. Those trips would be filled with information and conversation, infusing Nancy's imagination with the stories and creations of artists from around the world. With her Grandmothers encouragement, she quickly learned to sketch and paint on tiny canvases, and began to develop her own style of impressionist abstracts and designs. "It was the first time I remember feeling that I could be or do something worth being seen. Even though I felt invisible, I thought my paintings could become my little offering, and I could hide behind them."

Sneaking into her father's study when he was at work, Nancy began to discover and explore the art books and the biographies of Monet and Cassatt, visualizing herself escaping to Paris to study and start her own life as an artist. But all too often her father would criticize her work, telling her that she was wasting her time.

Nancy recalled when she went away to college, she did so with the "strong encouragement" of her father to get a degree in English. She followed his wishes, but also was able to enroll in an off-campus art class with her own money. Here her talent blossomed, and her work was noticed by a local art gallery owner, who offered to display her work for free. "I wanted so much to see my paintings up on that wall," she said, the longing still clearly there. "But it seemed like too big of a risk. If I succeeded, my father would find out, and I couldn't stand the idea of my dream being ripped away from me. It was easier to just walk away."

After Nancy married and her children were older, she decided it was a safe time for her to try painting again. Like her father, her husband thought her "new hobby was a frivolous undertaking," so she would set a clock during the day to devote some time to paint when she was alone in the house, and set an alarm because she didn't want to "waste too much time at it." She'd finish the painting, and then quickly paint over it since she didn't want anyone to see or judge her work. "It was just for me," she said.

Nancy's son, however, later discovered her artwork and took one of her paintings to school to show his art teacher. The art teacher connected Nancy with a friend who owned a local art gallery that offered her the opportunity to include a few of her paintings in their opening gala. Two years after that, Nancy is teaching at that same gallery and is now a prominent artist in the city of Boston.

So, here's how Nancy and I translated her story in terms of her life map of fear and love specifically to passion for art.

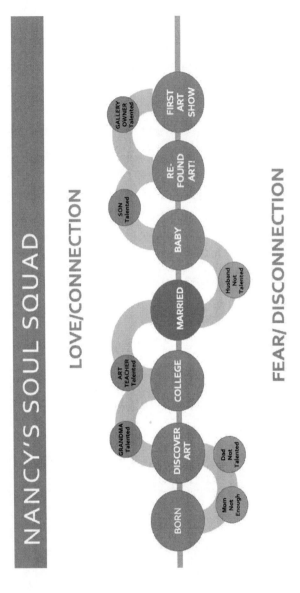

This is such a compelling story of how love and fear can mold one's self-esteem, and thereby influence the soul's purpose. But if you look at how the story unfolded, you can clearly see how each member of Nancy's squad offered her the opportunity to define her life's path. Can you see how all of those soul mates, including her father,

grandmother, son and art teacher helped mold her preferences and choices? And can you see how they could
potentially have done that from a "higher" place of love
planned to offer these opportunities to grow, before she
was born?

Seeing her lifemap laid out like this not only helped
Nancy validate her yearning to become an artist, it helped
her see how her parents and husband had sharpened her
desire to take action, even though their opinions activated
fear and doubt within her. She also shared that she later
discovered that her father, had also wanted to be an artist,
but had been "strongly encouraged" to become a doctor
by his father. And Nancy's mother, had met Nancy's father
in college...in art class! "This exercise really helped me not
only understand what I came to do, but also helped me
understand and forgive my parents, and see how they too,
abandoned their dreams to fear."

Here's the thing...as you look at your milestones, you will
always find the **recurrent fear themes almost always start
at some point in childhood.** It's the time when we are often
talked out of our talent by people who discouraged us
(usually out of their own feelings of fear and lack) and a
time when we don't have a voice to fight back. In Nancy's
case, she was taught at an early age that her love of art
was "bad" and while she continued to feel drawn to using
her gift, she did so in a way that was hidden and measured
(literally) by time.

Whenever those fears entwine with a talent or something
that you love, like Nancy's love of art, it is a clear "flag"

that this is something attached to your life's purpose. Pay attention to it!

Optimizing Your Super-Powers

OK, you have come exceptionally far...so I want to empower you with some magic. With all of the insights from above, you are no doubt seeing how your divine squad mates have assisted you in helping you define your preferences and life decisions. And while it may be challenging to steer your earthly boat with and around our human soul mates, we have a superpower at our fingertips that you can activate to help connect with divine guidance and help any time we need it.

This is the reason we have our angels and spirit guides as part of our Soul Squad. And we can connect with them anytime we need them. The key? You have to ask! Your angels and guides have been divinely appointed to be of service to you, but cannot intervene in your life without your consent. Free will, remember?

Here are some examples of times when our angels and guides can be of most help to us:

1. You want to pursue something you were always meant to do and need an affirmation that you are divinely supported.
2. You feel alone or isolated and you need a sign that you are not alone.
3. You've been through a traumatic experience and need divine support through the healing process.
4. You are going through a spiritual awakening and you need inspiration to help deepen your understanding of your calling and your place in the universe.

So how do you ask for help?

Here are some really easy ways to connect.

1. Sit in a quiet space or somewhere in nature. With a few deep breaths, close your eyes and gently invite your angels and guides to sit with you. Imagine them gently taking a place at your right and left...pleased and eager that you have called them into your circle.

2. Visualize them. What do they look like? Are they majestic beings of light? Do they seem familiar? Do you recognize any of them as deceased relatives or loved ones?

3. Ask for their names. You might be surprised that you get an immediate answer, and a name that is not familiar to you. My angel's name for example is "Laylou."

4. If you have a specific intention or question, ask them to send you a sign of clear confirmation. For example, one time I asked my angels to show me two elephants as a sign. (I thought that would be a really tough but undeniable sign that they were with me. And within two days, I was at a bookstore, at the cashier, and right in front of me were two – and only two – elephant change purses. It's so much fun when it happens!

5. Wait for feedback. If you don't feel you have an answer to your question immediately, thank them anyway, and let them know you understand that the answer will come and you'll watch for a sign that it's from them.

Your angels and guides are extremely clever, and have multiple ways of connecting with you. I love looking for these signs, as it is a powerful and undeniable reminder of the reality of our angels and guides at work.

Here's a few other signs to pay attention to:

1. **Signs in nature**: Butterflies, white feathers, rainbows, and "spirit animals" are all signs of angels on earth that are often communicated through the natural world.

2. **Signs around you**: Angel numbers (444,777,1111), pennies on the ground and license plates. Any time you see the same numbers repeated – like on a clock repeatedly such as 2:22, or 3:33, this is could be a sign of affirmation or alignment from your angels and guides.

3. **Signs within you:** Déjà vu, dreams, chills, flashes of light. Angels may find it easier to communicate with you when you are asleep or when your subconscious mind is in a more relaxed state, so pay attention to your dreams or sudden changes in your body like goose bumps that prompt you to pay more attention to what you are seeing, thinking or feeling.

I can't wait for you to play this wonderful game with your own angels and guides and feel the loving and real connection they have to you. This magical circle of unconditional love and guidance is there for you now and always. It is there to support you and your earthly soul squad on your amazing journey of this lifetime together.

In the next chapter, you'll learn how you've chosen this exact time and place to be born, to create and immerse yourself into this specific life adventure you have chosen.

Are you ready to learn more about the wonderous, wonderful you?

Onward!

SOUL GOODY BAG

Here are some resources mentioned in this chapter for you for further exploration:

Your Soul's Plan: Discovering the Real Meaning of the Life You Planned Before You Were Born by Robert Schwartz. Your Soul's Plan explores the premise that we are all eternal souls who plan our lives, including our greatest challenges, before we are born for the purpose of spiritual growth, showing that suffering is not purposeless, but rather imbued with deep meaning.

Ask Your Angels: A Practical Guide to Working with the Messengers of Heaven to Empower and Enrich Your Life by Alma Daniel, Timothy Wyllie and Andrew Ramer Ask Your Angels vividly chronicles how angels are currently reaching out to every one of us in a totally new way and how we can draw on their power to reconnect with our lost inner selves and to achieve our goals.

Lisa Nitzkin: Spiritual Medium and Intuitive Counselor: https://www.lisanitzkinmedium.com - Using her energy senses, Lisa is able to connect to the spiritual energy of the deceased and provide validating information about these individuals for her clients regarding past, present and future experiences. This practice, called readings, is meant to lovingly guide individuals on their spiritual path and to validate that after we die, our souls still remain.

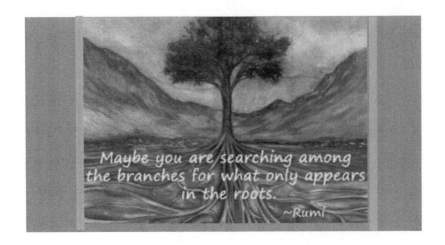

Maybe you are searching among the branches for what only appears in the roots.

~Rumi

CHAPTER 5

UNDERSTANDING YOUR ROOTS

On August 30, 1972, Wayne W. Dyer drove to Biloxi Mississippi with the "soul" intention to pee on his father's grave. At the time, he was a 32-year-old college professor at St. John's University. A series of synchronistic events led him to embark on a business trip that took him to the same town where his father, whom he had never met, was buried.

Jumping into the rental car at the airport, he found a business card taped to the seatbelt advertising the "Candlelight Inn" located in Biloxi. He acknowledged the coincidence that this hotel was located in the same town he was headed to, but when directed to the tiny, remote cemetery, he was stunned to learn that his father's grave was located on the grounds of the Candlelight Inn.

As Wayne approached the tiny plot on the peddler's field and saw his father's name on the marker, he flew into a rage allowing the anger of his lifetime to erupt from his soul. The years of living in poverty and foster care because his mother couldn't support him. His feelings of abandonment, confusion, loss, loneliness, and resentment, knowing his father was gone and had never once reached out for a word or a moment with his son.

But in the end, after his tirade of yelling, crying, shouting and demanding answers from the grave, Wayne finally fell silent and began to write. "As the hours pass," he writes, "I begin to feel a deep sense of relief, and I become very quiet. The calmness is overwhelming. I am almost certain that my father is right there with me. I am no longer talking to a gravestone but am somehow in a presence I cannot explain." Wayne decides he has said his peace and turns to leave. But as he gets back to his car, something stops him in his tracks. It was if he could feel his father's presence lingering there. That somehow, he had heard the grief and anger, and was still listening from the other side. The conversation, he sensed, was not quite finished.

So, instead of leaving, Wayne goes back to the gravesite. He speaks again, but now in words that he describes were very different. He is now talking to the *soul* of his father, the man who was the alcoholic, the man who died alone. At that moment, Wayne experiences a transformational moment of forgiveness from deep within his own soul. And his conversation with his father changes forever. "From now on," he says out loud. "I send you only love." In that moment of profound release, a miracle takes place. The power of the past, the power of the anger and the power of his childhood abandonment is gone. (ISCN p.146)

Within two weeks of that lifechanging moment, Wayne writes his first best-selling book, "Your Erroneous Zones" which he says, was virtually channeled from his soul. The book was the beginning of a writing and speaking career that spanned four decades. He has written over 40 books and influenced the lives of millions around the world.

As Wayne reflected on this lifechanging experience in his book "I Can See Clearly Now" he explains how looking back at all of his life's events showed him that there are teachers and teachings everywhere.

"I urge you to apply an unobstructed view to everything that has ever happened to you, and everyone who has ever come into your life," he writes. The events or people that show up in your life are not because of happenstance and coincidence. There is something right in front of you, staring you in the face, offering a choice to grab ahold and get on board to travel in a new direction, or to ignore it, and attribute it to nothing more than chance. As you adopt more of an 'I can see clearly now' attitude, you will look very differently at every aspect of your life." (ICSCN p. 357-358)

Each and every one of us has a lifetime of experience, but how often do we take the time to reflect back on how strong we really were, even in our mistakes and our everyday routines? How often do we take our circumstances as pure happenstance? Our so called "good and bad luck" as random experiences?

"Examine the major turning points in your life and look carefully at all of the so-called coincidences that had to arise in order for you to shift direction." Wayne continues. "At that moment you think of coincidence, you had a free will and you made a choice. At the same moment there was something much bigger than you, something you're always connected to, that was also at play. That something was setting up the details so you could fulfill the purpose you signed up for when you made the leap from Spirit to form, from nowhere, to now here." (ICSCN p.359)

This is the thinking that became the foundation of the book in your hands.

Understanding the Roots of Our Soul

Our human spirits are rooted in our emotional foundation. We are nurtured and nourished when we have access to earthly experiences that fill our hearts, minds and bodies to fuel our growth, our energy and our expansion. These are the roots of our source.

This chapter will invite you to step back in time and survey the environment that you were planted in. To take mental inventory of your early memories and experiences that formed the basis of you... to remember that spark of light that *is* you and the events and circumstances that accompanied your journey into this world.

This is the landing field from where your earliest intentions began. The soil in which you planted the seeds of your ideals and aspirations. This was the place that would activate your soul code...the marvelous, miraculous, ever-evolving you that is activated by every choice, interaction, and circumstance. Your soul code is activated though every experience that causes you to grow, expand, evolve and immerse your roots deeper into mother earth to flourish, thrive and prosper.

Within this code are the key building blocks of *who* we are, what we believe and *how* we interact on the planet.

Here is where you will layer on the situations and surroundings in your early life as you came to understand the world, to help you understand the "**WHAT's**" – meaning, those early circumstances such as religion, poverty, politics, health, finances, family dynamics and world events, that influenced your opinions, beliefs and impressions of where and how you lived. This was the foundation of your love and fear compass that helped you understand and navigate your path on the planet.

These lesser-known forces of our conscious and subconscious, many of which were formed at the earliest stages of life, can potentially be at the heart of what might be making you feel stuck, unsure, derailed, prone to procrastination, or less productive than you desire.

Going through your roots will uncover all of the interwoven threads in your human tapestry. And rather that pushing them underground or deep within, we will invite you to uncover them a bit, prune what you need, expose them to a bit of water (tears if you need) and sunshine, and give them the credit that they deserve for helping you grow into the majestic being that you are.

In this chapter you will:

- **Explore** the framework of how you grew –the outer and circumstantial influences of your **Mind** (culture, beliefs, ancestry), **Body** (your physical environment, wealth and processions) and **Spirit** (your inner world-your emotional experiences and relationships).
- **Define** what we mean by "Basic Needs" and how these have influenced our childhood, young adult experiences and ultimately who we are today.
- **Examine** how our astrological identities have helped shape and guide our path.
- **Take inventory** of our early Physical and Emotional Environments to better understand the roots of our experiences.

- **Release** any preconceived fears or judgements from the past and re-affirm our path to love over fear.

Another amazing layer in your exquisite tapestry is waiting to be revealed. Shall we?

Understanding Our Basic Needs

I've always been fascinated by the intersection of science and spirituality. When I was in school, we studied psychologist Abraham Maslow's hierarchy of needs, which was always illustrated in the form of a pyramid that painted a fairly rigid scientific picture of the essential things people needed to live. Maslow's theory suggested that people have a number of basic needs that must be met before people move up the hierarchy to pursue more social, emotional, and self-actualizing needs. Basically, the idea was "man cannot live by bread alone, but it all starts with the bread."

Maslow said, to live a so-called "self-actualized life," or to be fulfilled and do everything you are capable of, you need to satisfy every layer of the pyramid from the bottom to the top. At first, when you look at how the pyramid is built, it intuitively makes sense to index layers like food, shelter and safety as critically important components to the foundation of one's existence.

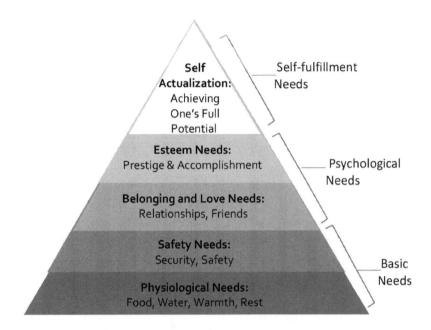

But while the layers themselves make sense individually, for me, they didn't add up collectively as a holistic pathway to wholeness. Even as a young adult, I knew that there were countless stories of those who were neither safe nor fed and yet were shining examples of self-fulfilled human beings.

Mother Theresa lived and served her community in the midst of poverty and violence, but was full and fulfilled within her mission of saintly service to others. Think of how many miraculous, inspiring lives have become living examples of the most accomplished beings who came from unimaginable poverty or emotional trauma. Oprah, Nelson Mandela, JK Rowling are just a few examples of those who started with nothing and worked their way to success. They did not require safety, security, or evidence of their accomplishments to lead and exude complete, fulfilled lives and ultimately inspire others.

They did, however, harness the power of their experiences of scarcity, physical abuse, illness and emotional trauma as their jumping off point to transformation and either consciously or subconsciously, made a choice to reach for love over fear.

Bloom Where You Are Planted

About the same time as I was learning about Dr. Maslow, my mother began posting signs all over the house, that were undoubtedly intended as subliminal psychological mind-control of her six growing offspring.

I remember rolling my eyes with annoyed distain, as the signs kept populating everywhere in the house, embossed with their perky flowers and pastel hearts.

"Bloom where you are planted," was the quote on the plaque above our dinner table.

"When life gives you lemons, make lemonade," was placed gingerly just above the telephone in the kitchen.

"Today only happens once, make it amazing," was just above our bathroom mirror.

All this not–so-subtle subliminal messaging created a very confusing picture. Should I make the best of whatever situation came my way? Or reach for the top of the pyramid?

The answer, of course, is both.

Your Earthly Fingerprint

When you first enter your body as a tiny infant, you are suddenly submerged into a tumultuous planetary melting pot of emotions, energies, events and experiences. And while you carefully selected your parents, where you would be living, and even the precise date and time of your birth, you are destined to slowly lose memory of your extreme wonderfulness, perfection and supreme power; the essence of your soul and your soul's intention for this lifetime.

We agree to this forgetfulness, as we have said, to help us better embrace our earth school of learning. And yet, the keys to these memories and intentions are always there for the finding, if we just look for them.

Maslow and my mother both got it right. Part of our work is to reach for the stars, that top of the pyramid...evolving always toward our full potential...to what we intended to become, do, achieve and give. But it is also about the **be-ing,** the immersing our full soul and spirit into the raw, naked and volatile earth toward everything thrown at us and done to us. Once we lean into our life circumstances, we are to pull up the nutrients of those unbridled experiences into our roots, standing full in our effervescing truth... and then to quite simply.... bloom.

How Your Astrological Chart Plays A Role in Your Roots

So, as we begin to trace our roots back to our beginnings, imagine that your life's plan was so intricate, so celestial, that your soul's DNA was actually mapped to the stars, and that it is all part of a stellar, spectacular plan we make ahead of our calculated landing on the planet.

Got your attention?

Earlier, I shared with you my story about the impact that an astrological reading had upon me as a thirteen-year-old girl, overwhelmed with the idea of choosing a career, feeling awkward about everything and good at nothing. The insights I received from that reading, literally filled my heart with hope, that there could be some meaningful contribution that I could make to the world...and that maybe, I was here to accomplish something of purpose.

Here's a conversation that I had with my grandfather, a well-meaning, loving, and very traditional father of seven boys. The "what do you want to be when you grow up" question always terrified me. Deep inside, I had an inkling of what I wanted to do, but I had no confidence. Any outward utterance of the idea that I wanted a job in television, seemed like a pompous, outlandish dream in 1975. And yet, when my Pop-Pop lovingly posed the life assessment question, I decided to test the waters.

Pop-Pop: "So, what are you thinking you want to do with your life Karen?"

Me: "I don't know Pop. I was thinking maybe a teacher (play it safe answer first) ...or...maybe.... (long pause) ...something in TV...? (best to not be too specific/ hold breath.)

Pop-Pop: "Hmm.... (really, really long pause) I think you should be a teacher. There are only seven TV channels, and it'll probably be really hard to get a job in TV."

I gave Pop-Pop credit...he didn't end that last sentence with, "because you're a woman," but I was disappointed in his answer. Even though I know he was trying to advise on a more secure route for my future, his response lacked confidence in me. The more inspiring follow-up would have been, "interesting choices...which one of those two jobs sounds more exciting to you?" or "you'll be good at anything you set your mind to, Karen."

So, when an astrologer, who didn't know me from a hole in the wall, said there was hope for me in the land of science, television and technology, I was thrilled, even though I had no idea those fields would eventually become my career.

That's when astrology became the shining star that I wanted to chase. It was hope. And I became obsessed with trying to learn more about it.

What Is Astrology: Your Soul's Chosen DNA

From the beginning of time, stars and planets have always inspired a sense of wonder.

Cultures, religions and civilizations looked skyward to understand seasons and weather pattens. Others looked for and found the face of the divine there.

There's a cosmic dance on the grand scale, and one on an intimate scale, going on for each of us. Astrology is the study of patterns and relationships — of planets in motion, our birth chart, synchronicity with others — and using that knowledge as a tool to understand our place in the universe.

When I first began my astrological quest, there weren't too many books on the subject. One pioneer that wrote multiple books on astrology was Linda Goodman. Quirky, hilarious, eccentric, she was the first astrologer to have a book on the New York Times bestseller list. She also lived the later part of her life in a self-professed haunted house in an old mining town in Colorado.

In her groundbreaking book, SunSigns, published way back in 1968, Linda set up a captivating definition of the science of reading the stars. "Our astrological natal chart is like a photograph of the exact position of all the planets in the sky at the moment of your birth." (SunSigns p.xix). "As you play the "Sun Signs" game, you'll be learning something very serious and useful: how to recognize your hidden dreams, secret hopes and true character...and how to really *know* the people you think you know. It's a happier world, when you look for the rainbows hidden inside them.... understanding the twelve sun signs will change your life." (Sun Signs xxiv)

And so, it did for me. Reading through her series of books that combined her own autobiographical relationships and experiments, with astrology, numerology, spells, lexigrams, ghosts and avatars, not to mention her personal recipe for physical immortality (thought transformation, leading to the achievement of cell regeneration) and chronicles of her days in Hollywood, she was a story of a woman with a well-lived life, that was clearly ethereally charged with her knowledge of the stars, science and metaphysical insights.

In the preface of her book "Star Signs" written in 1987, an ancient like wisdom, an outer-worldly knowing, shines through as she introduces the importance of astrology in her view of civilization:

> "...answers to all conceivable questions can be seen, even the proof of the validity, through a multiplicity of codes and signs beyond – yet inseparable from astrology. As unrelated to planetary influences as these prisms of knowledge may first appear, they nevertheless all initiative from the Luminaries (the Sun and Moon) and the stars of the planets. They are the Star signs of wisdom, awaiting your discovery." (SS xxv).

And so, they are.

Linda's books are given credit, like many of the others that came out in the 1980's for setting the spark to the New Age movement. Here, Linda nods to the growing enlightenment waking up the planet:

"It is good that humans are, at long last, beginning to realize who they really are – to recognize their own marvelous magical abilities... "Earthing's" are finally becoming dimly aware that they are in truth, spirits, imprisoned in flesh, "Body Temples" and afflicted with eons-old amnesia of each individual's true identity and birthright of divinity."

— (Linda Goodmans Star Signs p. xvii)

This is another one of those books that presents deep, ancient insights, that take time to absorb and understand, and yet I marvel at the depth of when she knew at the time, without any connection to the internet, or the connections to the knowledge we now have at our fingertips.

And while a journey with Linda through the stars, numbers, ancients puzzles and poetry can be a dizzying, bedazzling mind-blowing trip of life-inspiring learning proportions, she too held firm that our true power to navigate from the roots to the stars will be always found within our own true selves.

Real Truth, can be found in one place only – in every man's and woman's communion with an eternal Source of hidden Knowledge within – which each individual must seek and find for himself or herself. We may point out the path to others, but each must walk along that path alone, until every single "lost one" has made the whole journey – and all of us have finally reached the Light of full-born Wisdom at the end of the Way...where we began, a long-forgotten Time ago.

— (Linda Goodmans Star Signs p. xvii)

How wonderful that we have so many tools and teachers to help us as we look to both our roots and the stars to help light our way!

Stevie's Seeker Story: A Diagnosis Becomes A Destiny

Taking the time to have your chart read and to understand the basics of your natal numerology will provide you with an invaluable layer of insight into your roots, as well as a roadmap to help you navigate where to go from here.

Take my friend Stevie Knispel for example. Her seeker journey began with a life-threatening illness when she was just a teenager.

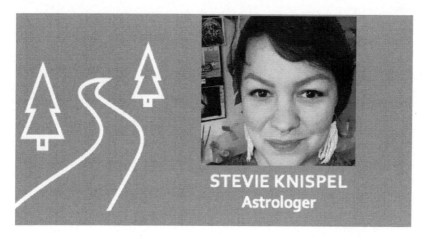

STEVIE KNISPEL
Astrologer

When I was 15, I found a lump on my ribs and was diagnosed with bone cancer. While I have ALWAYS been a person to look to the greater meaning of things and to connect to something unseen in order to guide me, in this moment, when I was just a freshman in high school, I was confronted with my entire existence.

While at first, I was scared of what I was facing, the worry faded as I knew those negative emotions would get me nowhere. My family inspired me to not take the path of fear. Instead, I felt a strong need to be strong and to choose love. I felt a need to use my perspective to look up above the uncertainty and choose gratitude for everything I had in my life. My family grew so much closer during this time. My mother and I, who had so been disconnected in my early teenage years, grew much closer. I was confronted with such intense unconditional love from her that it put everything into perspective.

I knew I had to choose love, and it was the only way out.

Going through that experience changed me in every way. My physical body changed, my spiritual and emotional body transformed. I knew that my energy, thoughts and my attitude would change the course of my life. My choices had an effect on those around me, those I loved.

I've taken that reminder with me ever since, and tried to live from a place of LOVE and not fear, where I choose gratitude and a higher perspective that knows all is well, and I am well.

That experience gave me the gift of knowing life is precious and that I'm here for a reason...to help others choose love.

Today, I am an Astrologer and I am blessed to help other people see themselves through a soul lens, through the lens of their own soul contract. Astrology has helped *me understand why I am the way I am and why we go through certain experiences in our lives. And it's my greatest pleasure to help others see that as well.*

Stevie's early life experience shows us a great example of how incredible challenges that are faced early in life can be the catalyst to facing fear, embracing love and courage, and finding our soul's purpose.

Identifying Root Causes: The Hidden Codes within Your Childhood

One way of deciphering this treasure trove of your soul's DNA can be unlocked by reviewing the formative years between the ages of 1 and 21. These are what are called the formative years, the time when our soul supper gets thrown into the pot to simmer...the meat (experiences), the spices (emotions), the flavors (the preferences) that will show us the true brew of our soul stew. It's the concoction we conjure...the recipe of our creation.... our slow simmer of evolution, based on our environment, where our winds of experience blow. The place where the buds and roots of your personality stem.

None of these experiences were random occurrences in time or space. Quite the contrary! Like your astrological birthdate, they were carefully chosen by you to help influence the foundation of your personality, your preferences, and yes, your loves and your fears.

In our next exploration, we're going to take a gentle look at some of those key life influencers that our friend Dr Maslow showed us in his life pyramid. These are early influencers that help till the soil that nurtures and infuses the ground where our human roots grow.

These are the circumstances in our **outer world** that impact our **inner world**.

What do I mean by that?

In addition to coming in and having our multi-sensory, personal interactions with our soul squad, we've also beamed down into a virtual melting pot of planetary events, activities and influences that impact our emotional and physical wholeness.

Our early environment and surroundings that we encounter as we embark on our earthly journey are like the water, sunshine and soil that fosters the tiny seedling of our soul. It has its own nugget of DNA –it's the intention of what it will become, with its own components and capabilities for physical manifestation and growth.

A sunflower seed will grow into a sunflower...an acorn into an oak tree. But no two are exactly alike.

Growth is influenced by its surroundings...where, when and how the seed is placed within the earth. Whether it gets enough sun or rain. If the dirt is deep or shallow, rich with nutrients or deficient, nested in a protected field, or trying to grow in a crack of pavement.

We come in with a plan for our life story, with our chosen set of people and opportunities for our growth, but the roots are our "setting:" the backdrop of current events that is going on around us. And it has so much influence on us. World hunger, political unrest, racial riots, a pandemic. How we shelter, our financial outlook, our sense of safety...all impact our **physical and emotional** health as an impression that helps us define our place on the planet.

These form the framework of your root belief system and have the most influence on your life between the ages of one and twenty-one.

We're now going to review and rank these memories and preferences that have impacted your root beliefs about yourself and the world. These, like your actual milestones and soul squad, have become intricate threads in your life's tapestry, interwoven with your adult preferences, emotions and beliefs.

To jump back into this portal in time, we'll approach this section within the framework of how **your mind** (view of the world, factual knowledge, habits, beliefs), **your body** (your physique, wellness, environment, wealth, processions) and **your soul** (inner world - emotional experiences, relation-ships) originated, evolved and expanded.

Ready to jump into the time machine?

Good. First, let's center and then we'll blast off.

Remembering Who We Were, And Still Are

For this Soulfirmation, take a moment to visualize yourself at age 7 or 8 years old. Focus on that little child's face. Feel the love that you have for that younger version of you...the empathy and appreciation for what it feels like to be a little person in a big world.

Take a moment to be back in the body of that little spirit of you.

- Where were you living?
- Who were the people that were part of your day-to-day experiences?
- What were some of your daily activities?
- Who were the influencers in your life? Your com-panions?
- What was going on in the world at the time?

Allow your current self to visualize and embrace that innocent, younger soul of you.

Appreciate the courage that it took for your little self to come forth knowing that your footsteps were heading in the direction of many earthly experiences that would be orchestrated for your highest good and soul's evolution.

You are, without question, a life warrior!

Breathe and absorb this deep understanding for a moment. Your innocence and experiences come together as you feel the multi-experiential, multi-emotional, multi-dimensional you.

Feel it all...thank the you who has taken this journey with such wisdom and courage. With every single step you have learned so much. You have done well because all of it is about simply taking the journey and doing your best with what you know.

When you are ready to begin, repeat the following affirmation.

 SOULFIRMATION #5

"I fearlessly set the intention to explore my past for the clues to my present.
I am safe to lovingly embrace my inner child
to explore the world of my younger self in all my innocence and openness,
before I was taught to question otherwise.
This is the me of my beginning
that will help me remember my map for the me of my future."

Repeat the affirmation as many times as you need to so you can fully get to a place of full allowing. Allow whatever thoughts, emotions, sensations, or feelings to come.

Breathe in deeply and hold it for as long as you can.
And then exhale deeply.
Repeat.
Good…. you are now in the life-flow.

LIFEMAPPING EXPLORATION #4:

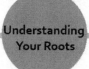

Understanding
Your Roots

Lifemapping Reminder: As we continue, the same guidelines apply:
1. Give yourself a time limit – 15 minutes is a good goal for this exploration.
2. As in our prior exercises, find a comfortable location for you to do this work.
3. Try not to overthink it.
4. Be gentle with yourself – if this becomes too emotional for one sitting, you can divide this exercise into parts, or come back when you are ready.

Ok, here is the process.

Step: 1: Rank:

- Starting with *your physical environment*, on a scale of 1, being very negative to 5 being very positive, rank how your felt about some of the key and basic needs in your life…your safety and security, your home, your health. For example, if your family had financial problems, or lived in a home that was in a dangerous area that caused you to be fearful at a young age, you might rank those as 1 or 2 on the negative scale. Or, if your home and finances didn't impact your thinking at all, you might give it a 3 or even 4 on the neutral or positive scale. If, however your home and finances were plentiful, and brought you joy and positive feelings, you might rank it "very positive' and tally it as a 5 in that column.

- Approach *your emotional environment*, in the same way. These are the aspects that impacted your psychological development...your self-esteem and feelings of worth, your relationship with your family and the outside world. If, for example, people in your home were judged or experienced religious or cultural bias and it made you feel angry, you might rank it as a 1 or 2 on the negative scale. Or if religious or cultural bias was part of your experience but it had no real impact, you might rank it as a 3 on your chart. If, however, this judgement or bias empowered you, and made you feel like you could make a positive difference in spite of this situation, you might give it a 5 on the positive scale.

Step 2: Evaluate:

- While not a requirement, it is helpful to add some notes after each section on what influenced the rank you chose. This will add valuable insights to this exercise later.

- It's also important to add that if one category was really positive at a young age and turned extremely negative at a later stage of your adolescent, this is a critical thing to note, as its impact on your emotional scale will be even more significant.

- As in all of these exercises, they are not intended to be precise...these are just ways of trying to fill in the layers of critical moments along your life's path to provide you with insight on the "what's" that influenced you on the early part of your journey.

- And, like all of the other exercises, do your best to look at these experiences as "other moments" that unfolded in your life's movie...without too much judgement of yourself, or the other people who may have played a role in these events. Remember, this is all about understanding the unfolding and what those key experiences are trying to show you.

Step 3: Tally:

- Add each column individually and then sum the total at the very bottom.

Now, it's your turn. Use the template on the next page for your exploration.

ROOTS EXPLORATION						
	Very Negative (1)	Negative (2)	Neutral (3)	Positive (4)	Very Positive (5)	Notes
PHYSICAL ENVIRONMENT						
Political/Environmental						
Home/ Living Environment/ Security						
Finances/Money						
Health/Illnesses						
School/Education						
Talents/Activities/Hobbies						
Body Image/Appearance						
EMOTIONAL ENVIRONMENT						
Religion/Spirituality						
Family/Relationships						
Freedom/Opportunity						
Death/Divorce/Abandonment						
Sexuality (Shame/Self-Esteem)						
Prejudice/Judgement/Bullying						
Opinion of Self						
TOTALS						Total -

OK, Now for the Big Reveal!!

Reading Your Root Scale: When you tally up your numbers of your roots assessment, what overall message does it convey to you about your earlier years?

60-70 – Very Positive/Love Based
49-59 – Positive/Love Based

38-48 – Neutral (Neither overly negative or positive)
26 -37 – Negative/Fear Based
14 -25 – Very Negative/Fear Based

The important thing to note here is that your score is not reflective of the **quality** of your childhood or young adult life. This isn't a **judgement** call of "good" or "bad" or getting a high or low score. It is merely a reflection of the environmental landscape you encountered as you beamed yourself down on this planet, and your point of "emotional reference" to it.

Every life experience is only equal to the emotional reaction to it, regardless of how the world defines it. Meaning, you get to decide how important, or devastating or non-eventual each of these situations were based on your own experience... not how the world may evaluate or judge it. A child living in poverty with a single mother working full-time, for example, can still feel completely loved, safe, and prosperous, while a child coming from an affluent, two parent household can feel disconnected, discouraged and depressed.

The most noteworthy part of the exercise for you is that the **lower the score**, and the places you felt the most fearful and negative, are the **places to now consider shining your light.**

For a moment, take a look at those places with the "1's" and "2's". Are there opportunities for forgiveness there? For yourself? For others? Might this be a time for you to let go of that fear, blame, anger and shame about that situation? To release that memory from your little body, and innocent heart, knowing you did the very best you could at that time, and now re-record over it from the perspective of your older wiser self, with a newfound understanding of the lesson it offered you?

Yes, this is big work. Just sit with this for a minute. While it can be painful to look back on these fearful moments, our early lives offer us powerful clues to some of the lessons we have come here to learn. And for many of us, we simply haven't gotten the report card reflecting the incredible students we are, and the resilient, awe-inspiring teachers that we have become. Take Caroline for example.

CAROLYN'S STORY: Rewriting the Past

Those are the words written by Carolyn in her journal after doing the root exercise. She read them aloud to our little group, surprising even herself as she shared them. Exquisite poetry channeled from within.

"I'm not sure where that came from," she said quietly.

Ah, but how eloquent the heart can be when it wants to speak its truth.

Carolyn didn't come to my Lifemapping workshop willingly. Her daughter Vanessa had signed her up and talked her into it as a way of spending some "mother-daughter time" together.

I loved the sweetness with how Vanessa "lured" her mother into our session. "I love my mom so much...she's one of the most giving people you will ever meet. But I don't really know her. I mean I know *about* her, her life experiences and all that, but I want to know *who* she is on the inside. It's a piece of her that I hope she can share with me."

Carolyn had just celebrated her sixtieth birthday. Her husband and four children had taken her on a cruise to the Bahama's, something that had been on her bucket list for her lifetime. They also presented her with a beautifully embossed photobook that was full of pictures of her childhood growing up in Atlanta. "It brought back memories of things I had forgotten," Carolyn said, her voice trailing off.

Vanessa added context. "Mom had a tough childhood, and just recently shared with us some of the stories of what she went through. It was...a lot. The book really helped her release some of those emotions, which is why I think this class will help her sort through some of the meaning of those early times in her life."

With that context from Vanessa, it was interesting to see how Carolyn approached her milestone and soul squad exercises. Most of the key events that she listed on her timeline occurred after high school.

Carolyn didn't realize this until we reached the root exercise. "It's so interesting," she said, "I haven't thought about that early part of my life, since I didn't view it as a time of real accomplishment with events worth remembering. I didn't think of those times as hard. It was just what I knew it as ... my "normal."

But it was **anything but** normal.

Carolyn grew up in downtown Atlanta in the early sixties, the daughter of a single mom, living in a low-income neighborhood with her three siblings. It was an era of racial upheaval, of riots and demonstrations, with lots of police unrest. It was a scary time to be an African American living in the south.

Carolyn remembered the moldy walls and bad ventilation in the apartment triggering severe asthma attacks and being afraid that she'd have to go to the hospital, which her mother couldn't afford. She recalled the sense of anger and abandonment she felt when her father left them, and the fear that she'd be put in foster care or homeless if something happened to her mother. She thought about the night she fought off a sexual attack by a neighbor, never telling anyone because she thought it was her fault, and didn't want to call attention to her family.

But she also remembered her love for family, her church, and the choir that helped her find her voice.

Now that she could look back with her adult eyes on her young life, she had a new appreciation for all of the challenges she faced. With Caroline's permission, I've shared her Roots Assessment as an example.

ROOTS EXPLORATION Carolyn						
	Very Negative (1)	Negative (2)	Neutral (3)	Positive (4)	Very Positive (5)	Notes
PHYSICAL ENVIRONMENT						
Political/Environmental	1					We were living near the Atlanta riots and demonstrations. Lots of police unrest.
Home/ Living Environment/ Security	1					Our house was in the low renter's district of Atlanta in a dangerous neighborhood. We had break-ins all the time.
Finances/Money	1					My mom worked 2 jobs to make ends meet. Money was scarce.
Health/Illnesses	1					We couldn't afford doctors, so I was always worried about getting sick. I had many allergies triggered by mold.
School/Education		2				I liked school, but I had to work at it. I never felt very smart.
Talents/Activities/Hobbies					5	I loved singing with my friends in the choir. I was told I was very good!
Body Image/Appearance		2				I was definitely not the prettiest girl. I wished that I could have gotten braces.
EMOTIONAL ENVIRONMENT						
Religion/Spirituality					5	I loved being at church and singing in the choir. I had a strong belief in God which helped me though a lot.
Family/Relationships				4		I was very close to my mom and my grandmother and siblings.
Freedom/Opportunity		2				I never felt safe to go too far from home, and I didn't qualify for the financial aid for college.
Death/Divorce/Abandonment	1					My Dad left when I was seven. I always worried that my mom would die or leave us like he did, and I would have to go into foster care.
Sexuality (Shame/Self-Esteem)		2				I was nearly attacked by a neighbor when I was 14. I didn't tell anyone because I thought it was my fault.
Prejudice/Judgement/Bullying	1					I grew up in the 60's. It was a scary time to be African American in Atlanta.
Opinion of Self			3			I know I did the best I could with what I was given. I have always tried to be a good person.
TOTALS	6	8	3	4	10	Total - 32

Carolyn was wide eyed as she looked at her roots exploration for the first time.

"I'm so glad that I went back and looked at that time in my life again," Carolyn said. "I realize now that I was stronger that I realized, and those experiences helped set the course of my life."

Indeed, they did!

When Carolyn left Atlanta, she put herself through community college. She went on to raise her children with her loving husband, in a beautiful, safe suburban town in NJ, ultimately becoming an OBGYN nurse practitioner in a lower income community. "Thankfully, my Mom was able to live with us through the last years of her life," Carolyn added, "which helped me return the care and love she offered to us after working so hard all those years."

Looking back on these memories also helped amplify Carolyn's sense of pride that she could now see in her accomplishments. Those fearful beginnings helped teach her bravery and tenacity, which ultimately led to reaching for a life of love, and of giving back to both her mother and her community.

Vanessa summed it up best. "Those growing pains led mom from being fearful, to fearless. And now she's the most fearless person I know. And now I know why!"

"That's true," Carolyn laughed in agreement, "That is very true."

And the truth shall set you free.

Carolyn's beautiful story shows us that sometimes we can overlook, even take for granted, the badges of our bravery. These feats of honor that we achieve when we are still very little, vulnerable people. But it is in those years that we haven't been talked out of who we are. Not yet. And it's all there if we try to remember.

You many feel, as Caroline did, that it may not be comfortable to take that time machine back to those early years of life. And it's perfectly fine if you just want to quickly take mental inventory of these events and not tally up the numbers of how they impacted you on the fear and love scale. That's ok, because, I'll bet you already know it anyway.

The last part of this exercise is to take a moment and log your "key takeaways." These are just **3 things** you may have learned about your younger self that you didn't already include in your initial milestones exercise.

Here's Carolyn's as an example:

ROOTS EXERCISE: KEY TAKEAWAYS:

LOVE:
1. My Singing/Friendships = Love of Belonging
2. My Church/Choir = Love of God/Spirituality
3. My Mom/Grandma = Love of great Mothers/ strength

FEAR:
1. My Dad leaving =Church/Choir = Fear of Abandonment
2. Living in Poverty = Fear of not having enough
3. Minority and Prejudice = Fear of Judgement

What Did You Learn?

The intention of this exercise was to separate you from the specific events and people associated with your milestones, and instead focus on the physical and emotional environment surrounding all your beginnings.

For the last piece of this exercise, I invite you to find a photo of yourself as a younger child, say 7 or 8 years old, and take a deep, loving look at that earlier version of you. Write a note to your younger self from your now older self. Remind him or her that their hopes and dreams are still safe and appreciated and tucked away even now. Remind your younger self that you appreciate them, just as they are. Ask them about their hopes and dreams...their favorite friends, teachers and toys. Tell them that they are amazing. That they are strong and beautiful and brave. That they are more than enough.

And sign the letter with love, "from your higher self." And don't forget to add the P.S. "Everything will be just fine, because I can see clearly now."

And so, it is, and will continue to be so, because you are, dear, wonderful, beautiful, soul child, ever so much more than enough!!

More than enough – indeed! Let's finish this chapter with a quote from our now kindred guru, Linda Goodman, to tie a bow around our thoughts on the powerful wonders we are. These are the final sentences from StarSigns:

> "Do you see the wonderful thing this proves? It proves that you are already magical, and have been since you were born... you are all gods and goddesses, possessing great powers you have too long forgotten.
>
> Now that you have the code, what are you waiting for? There must be many other miracles you've been dreaming about. Stop dreaming and go right ahead... manifest them! Abracadabra! (SS p.466)

And "Abracadabra," as we know, in the magic form and otherwise, means, "so I say, so shall it be."

So, viola! Let us move on to Chapter 6 – and manifest the magic in "Decoding your Story!"

 SOUL GOODY BAG

Here are some resources mentioned in this chapter for you for further exploration:

- **I Can See Clearly Now by Dr. Wayne W. Dyer** - In this revealing and engaging book, Wayne shares dozens of events from his life, from the time he was a little boy in Detroit up to the present day. In unflinching detail, he relates his vivid impressions of encountering many forks in the road, taking readers with him into these formative experiences. Yet then he views the events from his current perspective, noting what lessons he ultimately learned, as well as how he has made the resulting wisdom available to millions via his lifelong dedication to service

- **Sun Signs by Linda Goodman** - Find out what's really happening in your life and the lives of those around you. Amaze your friends and yourself with your insight into their most hidden characteristics. Learn all this and much, much more from the world-famous astrologer who has helped millions find their way to happiness, love, and profit by studying the sun signs.

- **Star Signs by Linda Goodman** - Here, in her most personal book yet, Linda Goodman, America's premier astrologer, has written an enlightening and remarkably accurate guide to help you discover all the powers you possess. How can you achieve financial freedom and financial security? Which holistic healing methods really work? What hidden meanings can be found in numbers, words, and deja vu? How can music, color and crystals be used to improve your body and your mind? With her usual compassion, wit, and perception, Linda Goodman broadens the horizons of astrology to help you on your way to health and happiness.

- **Stevie Knispel – Astrologer - farmhousemoon.com.** Stevie's goal is to break down Astrology and give practical tools to help guide you on your spiritual journey and to help people come alive in their own skin. These tools help empower individuals and promote growth and development. Stevie loves helping mothers and fathers understand their children through their birth charts thus promoting a culture of compassion within the family. She's studied evolutionary, archetypal, esoteric and shamanic astrology. Her brilliant cumulation of those practices-her own special gift- has proven to be transformative and effective for those who apply her methods.

- **The Theory of Human Motivation by Abraham H. Maslow: Maslow** introduced the world to a new way of looking at the drivers of human behavior, growth and motivation. In essence, this book examines a profound question- what are our basic needs and what causes us to desire self-fulfillment and to become everything that one is capable of becoming?

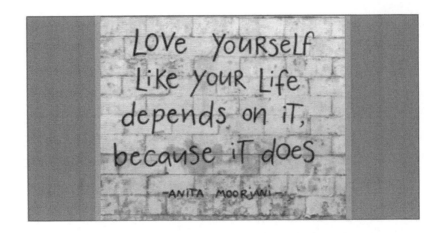

Love yourself
like your life
depends on it,
because it does
—ANITA MOORJANI—

CHAPTER 6

DECODING YOUR STORY

Once upon a time, a young boy named Santiago set off on a quest to travel the world, and learn about the science of turning lead into gold. Before he departs on his epic journey, he visits a gypsy fortune teller to help him interpret a recurring dream he's been having about finding a buried treasure, in the hopes that she can help him discover where it's hidden.

The woman interprets the dream as a prophecy, telling the boy that he will discover riches at the Egyptian pyramids, but that he will need to go on a great adventure to find the treasure he is seeking. She gives Santiago a hint that the quest he will be undertaking will be the great journey to find himself.

"You came so that you could learn about your dreams," the wise old woman tells Santiago, "And dreams are the language of God. When he speaks in our language, I can interpret what he has said. But if he speaks in the language of the soul, it is *only you who can understand*."

This is, of course the beginning of the great story "The Alchemist" by Paulo Coelho, that tells the epic adventures of Santiago, a shepherd boy who travels the world in search of his treasure. Santiago's journey shares the essential wisdom of listening to our hearts, learning to read the signs along life's path, and, above all, following our dreams.

Throughout his adventures, the boy encounters many obstacles that test his bravery, and he soon realizes that he must follow his heart no matter how difficult the journey becomes. He learns to use this inner guidance as a personal compass to overcome fear and to never lose hope when faced with adversity. He learns to overlook the influences and opinions of society and to continue his journey onward no matter what.

When Santiago finally comes face-to-face with the great and powerful Alchemist, who will teach him how to turn lead into gold, the great wizard affirms the importance of Santiago fulfilling his own personal quest, but also his role in making a great contribution to the world. "No matter what he does," the Alchemist says to Santiago, "every person on earth plays a central role in the history of the world. And normally he doesn't know it."

At the end of the story, Santiago discovers that the great treasure he has been seeking is buried beneath the very tree where he had fallen asleep and had his original dream. He fulfills the prediction of the Alchemist who told him, "wherever your heart is, there you will find your treasure. You've got to find the treasure, so that everything you have learned along the way can make sense."

And so it is with you. You too have treasure within you, and it has been there all along.

Welcome to Chapter 6. Where you will discover yours.

Your Hero's Journey

If I were to Lifemap Santiago's journey of key milestone, it would probably go something like this:

1. Has dream
2. Follows dream
3. Gets lost
4. Gets beaten up
5. Finds hero
6. Follows the hero's advice
7. Gets beaten up again
8. Finds his way back home and discovers treasure.

And I'd be willing to place a bet, you'd feel your own hero's journey has been similar, maybe with the exception of number 8?

Ah, but fear not...your treasure has a treasure map!! And we are about to put in into your hands.

In the last few chapters, you've jumped back into the time machine to really look at the key moments in your life:

1. **The When's:** Your key life **Milestones** and how they impacted you
2. **The Where's:** Your **Lifebeat** and the choices you made between love and fear
3. **The Who's:** Your **Soul Squad** and what they taught you
4. **The What's:** Your **Roots** and the founding belief system

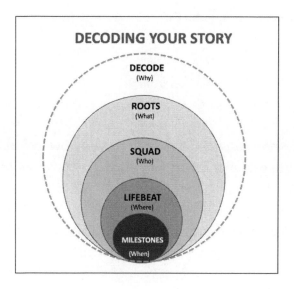

In this chapter, we'll go through your milestones and decipher their real meaning of love and fear in your life. This will help you begin to see the story of your own personal quest, and answer some of your great big questions about the **"WHY's"** – and what your milestones, your squad, your roots, have all been here trying to teach you. You will see and trace the steps that have made up your own hero's journey.

This is where you will begin to lay out the wholistic look at your life's purpose...by taking seemingly two very disparate experiences and laying them side by side for a brand-new meaning:

Experience 1: Our Love Path:

- Who you came to be
- What you came to teach
- What you need to do more of/expand/increase in your life experience

Experience 2: Our Fear Path

- What you came to work on
- What you need to release
- What you need to decrease in your life experience

This is the exercise that will show you how to further map the route you have taken to understand two key things – what you've come to **teach** and what you've come to **learn**. Yup, you've signed up for both.

Like Santiago's treasure discovery at the end of his quest, this is the place that will also bring you back to where you started – to decipher the meaning of your past from where you are at this present moment. This will help you to better understand the meaning of your journey, to best determine where to go from here.

This is the big stuff... where all of your hard work comes together, to help begin to paint the soul portrait of you.

Shall we begin?

Setting our Intention:

Before we get into the next few exercises, let's "do what we do," by setting our intention:

 SOULFIRMATION #6

"I set my intention
to offer gratitude for each and every one of my doubts and fears....
They are my team of life companions
as I venture off on my own quest to discovery why I'm here...
offering me choices to better know myself,
what I've come to do, to find, and what I have come to understand.
Love and Fear are friend and foe...
my path to know along my journey to grow."

LIFEMAPPING EXPLORATION #5:

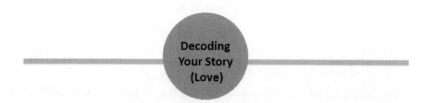

I like to refer to this section as "My Top 20 Hit List…" This is where we'll take a quick inventory of our map milestones to shine a loving light on our highest loves and our lowest fears. This is where you will begin to decode your story.

The key to this exploration is to **look at what those experiences might have taught you**, and put them in the context of your thoughts, beliefs and opinions about the "YOU" inside you.

In this exercise, you'll identify each love and fear milestone and create an **"I am" identity statement** for how that experience makes you feel or what it taught you about yourself.

> For example, if you stated that one of your **love milestones** was *going to college*, perhaps it made you feel like **"I am smart,"** or **"I am full of potential."**

> If, on the other hand, one of your **fear milestones** was **dropping out of college,** perhaps it made you feel like **"I am not smart enough"** or **"I am a failure."**

The reason we are going to take a look at your milestones through this lens of the "I am" is because this is the voice that we all have inside of our heads, that judges all our experiences and behaviors. This is our inner self that tells us the "story of who we are." The voice that sums up each experience, gives it and us a thumbs up or a thumbs down, and tells us who we are as a result of what we've done. This is our inner voice of fear or love which, in turn, communicates a feeling of love or light. This is the very thread we need to follow to understand our purpose.

Be not afraid...this may sound like a roller coaster ride... but I promise you...once you face both the fab and fierce, your power will be to see the version of you that might be hidden just outside your light in the shadows.

Lifemapping Reminder: Before we start, a reminder of our grounding rules.

1. Give yourself a time limit – 15 minutes is a good goal for this exploration.
2. As in our prior exercises, find a comfortable location for you to do this work.
3. Try not to overthink it.
4. Be gentle with yourself – if this becomes too emotional for one sitting, you can divide this exercise into parts, or come back when you are ready.

Part One: Decoding our Love Milestones:

Let us begin where we should always begin...**with LOVE**.
Here is the process:

Step 1: Identify – Go back to your life milestones **on page ###**– the ones you labeled "LOVE" – these are the ones that uplifted you...that made you feel valued, connected and joyful. Remember that person who was going through that experience.

Step 2: Evaluate - What are the takeaways about yourself that shine through and show you your essence...the light that is you.

Here is an example of how to "flip" your love milestones into "I am" statements.

Milestones	"I am" Statement
I started my own business	I am innovative, creative, and brave
I put myself through college	I am resilient, responsible and persistent
I married my best friend	I am loving, faithful, kind, and committed
I traveled to Peru with my church	I am a humanitarian, I am giving
I had a baby	I am selfless, a giver and a teacher

Here's a few tools to help you phrase your "I am" statements:

- How do you feel?
- What did it teach you about you?
- Did it make you feel connected or disconnected to your soul's purpose?

Step 3: Activate - Write out your I AM statement in the form on the next page– add as many as you want to your sheet. If you aren't comfortable creating 20 different "I am" statements, that's ok. You can also repeat the same "I am" statement if you feel similar experiences evoke the same feeling or emotion over and over again. You can also take a look ahead at my list on page 92, if you need some ideas to get you started.

Step 4: Reflect - When you have completed your list, take a few extra minutes to capture in your journal how these "I am" statements feel for you.

- Do they surprise you?
- Do they help you remember anything about yourself that you may have forgotten?
- Do you believe the "I am" statement?
- What could that role of that milestone be in your life?

Use the space below and begin.

THINGS I LEARNED FROM MY LOVE MILESTONES
1.
2.
3.
4.
5.
6.
7.
8.
9.
10.
11.
12.
13.
14.
15.
16.
17.
18.
19.
20.

Welcome to the Self-Love Shack Baby!

Alright … well done!! How about a big inhale here as you drink in all the love that's written on this page! Read through these statements out loud if you can.

Do you recognize, and are you willing to accept that beautiful-bright-boundless-source-energy- light that is you??!

Yeah, drink in that sunshine sweetie. It's yours and you earned every ray of light in that shower. Your sweet "I am's" are all that you have come to be and give. YES! This is the you, YOU came to be… this is YOU living your life's purpose! See yourself as the powerful, amazing, accomplished BAD ASS that you ARE!

This is a page that needs to be clipped and printed for you to look at every day because it is your soul, looking back at you!

Just for reference, I'll share my own Decoding My Milestones Top 20 List with you here.

THINGS I LEARNED FROM MY LOVE MILESTONES

1.   I am strong
2.   I am a seeker
3.   I am spiritual
4.   I am smart
5.   I am intuitive
6.   I am compassionate
7.   I don't give up/ am resilient
8.   I am caring
9.   I am courageous
10. I am always giving my best
11. I am a doer/create big goals
12. I am inspired
13. I am good at following my instincts
14. I am a learner
15. I am an inspirer
16. I am an explorer
17. I am a survivor
18. I am powerful
19. I am grateful / appreciative
20. I am an uplifter

When I look back at the milestones of my life where I was reaching for Love/Connection, they tell the story of my life as a seeker, almost from the beginning.

Even from my earliest childhood memories, I can see how choosing a childhood living with a spiritually open mother and grandmother opened me up to looking for meaning in things seen and unseen.

How venturing off to a distant college nurtured my curiosity as a seeker, my desire to learn new things both spiritually and intellectually, and of reaching for new adventures of exploration and expansion. How being a single mother and remarrying were acts of both survival and courage. How nurturing a child through cancer taught me to never quit, and to be both perseverant and resilient. Even how saying yes to running the Boston marathon (which I will share more about later) showed that I was willing to take risks and set big goals for myself.

Today, as I re-review my own list of these loving "I am" statements about my life, it refills me still. I can literally feel the inner light that is me shine through in these statements. I know they are "me" at my soul-level. They are my "Truth" – what I have on the inside to share and teach with the world. They also give insight into who I was created to be.

I hope that yours fills you with a similar grace and purpose and inspires you just like Santiago:

> "When you are loved," said Santiago "You can do any-thing in creation. When you are loved, there's no need to understand what's happening, because everything happens within you." (The Alchemist p.132)

Letting Your Inner Light Shine

Before we begin our next exercise, I want to share some observations from my beautiful friend, and Lifemapper, Katherine, who is both a deep soul-ful seeker as well as a profound spiritual teacher in her own right. She was partic-ularly moved by assessing the messages she received from her fear and love milestones, and the messages they showed her looking back at her life's path. Hers is another story of how her life-changing moment of facing her deepest fear, led to a personal transformation that revealed her purpose.

KATHERINE'S STORY: Lighting Up A New Path to Love

"Love is my most aligned path that allows my inner flow of myself to come forward as the love that I AM...to create a fulfilling life from the inside out."

My life-changing moment was, unfortunately, a broken heart. My then husband announced he was leaving me after a 15-year journey that had created our "dream life." I was truly devastated, really scared and felt like a failure. My mind, body, spirit and heart were in so many pieces that I could not see or feel how I would survive this fracture within me.

And then after some time had passed , I was processing some of these feelings... And I felt "it" happen. I was broken open to go deeper, my soul created an opportunity to go deeper within. This was an invitation, and opening to a journey further inside myself, my heart. To see and feel all that i tdidn't know or had feared about myself... My choices... My life. I began asking myself those really big questions.....how did I get here? Who am I? Where do I go from here? What is my purpose?

I was in so much fear of all those questions, and to face the unknown, but honestly I had nothing more to lose. I was inspired by my fear to dive deeper and find the answers. Another inspiration was the love around me. my family and friends that showed so much love to me when I was heartbroken. The love created a softening, a flow, a freedom, a strength that held steady...... connected me to myself and others. that love showed me how to stay open and receive, because I deserve to receive love....not just give it. That was a huge shift for me since I was an endless Giver....to the point of depletion. I was learning to allow myself to truly receive at a depth I never experienced before.

It was when I chose to face my fears, open up to receiving love, not just give it, that my courage to take the journey from a broken heart to an open heart began. This journey offered a lot of forgiveness to myself, as well as others. And a re-remembrance of me began to emerge...of who I truly was. I felt empowered to choose my truth and express it.

Within this expression is my life's purpose of helping others to remember who they truly are as well and supporting them in expressing it. I began to speak the Language of Light, a memory within all of us that we are love expressed creators, source energy, multi-dimensional beings in flow and everything we need is already within us. This remembrance of me as a source energy, a multidimensional being of love, in flow is answering all of my questions and creating new areas for me to explore.

Lifemapping brought forth awareness of how and why I chose my life's path. It clearly showed me how and why the fear-based decisions took me off my path of alignment with myself/soul and how and why my love-based decisions kept me in alignment and brought me back to self/soul alignment. Going forward with the enlightenment of my Life Mapping work, I now make decisions from my own self-love that are most aligned with my path. This method of deciding my destiny allows the flow of me to come forward as the love that I AM and creates a life fulfilled from the inside out.

Katherine's story shows the power of taking the Lifemapping journey to carefully look at each gift we are given, even in our pain and sorrow, as an opportunity to learn more about ourselves...to grow deeper...to open up ourselves to life even more.

Let's take a look at how embracing our fear milestones can be a gift in helping us explore, grow and heal in ways that bring us ultimately even closer to love.

LIFEMAPPING EXPLORATION #5 – Part 2

Decoding Your Story (Fear)

So, as we looked at LOVE life-milestones that took the outward action of reaching toward something that made us feel good/light/empowered on a soul level...the same is true of our fear-driven actions, except that those come from our disempowered self. These situations tend to be the ones where we hide our light under a bushel, and hide in the shadows of the places where we feel "less than" or disconnected from ourselves. Love is light. Fear is darkness.

In almost every case, this negative self-talk comes from the EGO, which Wayne Dyer used to say was "**E**dging **G**od **O**ut." Entire books have been written about the role of the ego, which some confuse with the idea of being "self-centered" or "full of it." In virtually every case, EGO is all about fear. It measures us against others. It loves to spread ideas of comparison and inadequacy. When you feel like you are "not enough," you are living in the space of EGO. EGO is the thing that tries to discourage us from seeing, doing and being what we came here to be.

It is the voice that tries to extinguish our light.

But here's the thing.

When you look at the milestones that have caused or inflicted fear in your life, or those situations where you might have made fear-based decisions, try to do so by keeping a tiny flashlight of love illuminated on your heart.

Because I guarantee in each case, if you can again pull yourself out of yourself and see the situation as an observer, you will find that the only failure or disappointment in that experience is the lack of love you had in that moment **for yourself**.

Shall we try this theory on for size?

Let us begin:

STEP 1: Identify – Go back to your life milestones – the ones you labeled "FEAR" – these are the ones that disempowered you...that made you feel undervalued, disconnected, disappointed. Take a moment, and lovingly remember that person who was going through that experience.

STEP 2: Evaluate - What are the takeaways about yourself that were shadows, imprints or experiences that dimmed the light within you.

Here is an example of how to translate your fear milestones into "I am" statements.

Milestones		"I am" Statement
I was fired from my job	⟶	I am worthless, irresponsible
My husband left me	⟶	I am unattractive, unlovable
I have cancer	⟶	I am sick, dying
I dropped out of college	⟶	I am not smart enough
I was abused as a child	⟶	I am weak and ashamed

Here's a few tools to help you phrase your "I am" statements:

- How do they make you feel?
- What did it teach you about you?
- Did it make you feel connected or disconnected to your soul's purpose?

STEP 3: List - Write out your I AM statement in the form below– adding as many as you want to your sheet. Again, if you aren't comfortable creating 20 different I am statements, that's ok. And like in the earlier Love exercises, you can also repeat the same "I am" statement if you notice that some experiences evoke the same "I am" feeling or emotion over and over again. You can also take a look ahead at mine if you need some ideas to get you started.

THINGS I LEARNED FROM MY FEAR MILESTONES
1.
2.
3.
4.
5.
6.
7.
8.
9.
10.
11.
12.
13.
14.
15.
16.
17.
18.
19.
20.

STEP 4: Reflect - When you have completed your list, take a few extra minutes to capture how these "I am" statements feel for you. (And yes, these will feel yuckier than the Love statements in the previous exercise.)

- Do they surprise you?
- Do they help you remember anything about yourself that you may have forgotten?
- Do you believe them?

Every fear, failure and disappointment is an opportunity to begin again.

These "I am's" are harder to look at and share, aren't they? Their frequency, or the energy that they have in your heart, feels very different, doesn't it? When I went through this Lifemapping experience myself, I realized that these fear-based judgements made me feel disempowered, less than...unworthy. And if I'm truthful, these are also the perceptions or my interpretation of what I imagined others thought about me. It made me feel like a fraud in my own life, or like I was trying in fact to hide behind my life in the shadows of the unseen.

THINGS I LEARNED FROM MY FEAR MILESTONES

1. I am a harsh judge of myself
2. I am not smart enough
3. I am not good enough
4. I am fearful
5. I am full of self-doubt
6. I am useless
7. I am not brave
8. I am afraid of confrontation
9. I am not confident
10. I am not a good person
11. I am afraid of being judged
12. I am afraid they will see through me
13. I am afraid to fail
14. I am too attached to success and outcome
15. I am afraid of speaking my truth
16. I am quick to blame myself
17. I am too nice
18. I am not strong enough
19. I am different
20. I am selfish

You may not feel empowered at the moment, but take another deep breath, because I promise you that you will find magic on the next page.

An amazing thing happened to me when I compared my two lists. Are you ready for the big reveal?

LIFE MILESTONES: STEP 3 — Love & Fear & Self

And the moment of truth...

Now that you've made your list of both your fear and love milestones, take a moment and put them side by side. I'll show you mine as an example.

So, this is where a lot of my "ah ha" moments came up.

THINGS I LEARNED FROM MY LOVE MILESTONES	THINGS I LEARNED FROM MY FEAR MILESTONES
1. I am strong	1. I am a harsh judge of myself
2. I am a seeker	2. I am not smart enough
3. I am spiritual	3. I am not good enough
4. I am smart	4. I am fearful
5. I am intuitive	5. I am full of self-doubt
6. I am compassionate	6. I am useless
7. I don't give up/ am resilient	7. I am not brave
8. I am caring	8. I am afraid of confrontation
9. I am courageous	9. I am not confident
10. I am always giving my best	10. I am not a good person
11. I am a doer/create big goals	11. I am afraid of being judged
12. I am inspired	12. I am afraid they will see through me
13. I am good at following my instincts	13. I am afraid to fail
14. I am a learner	14. I am too attached to success and outcome
15. I am an inspirer	15. I am afraid of speaking my truth
16. I am an explorer	16. I am quick to blame myself
17. I am a survivor	17. I am too nice
18. I am powerful	18. I am not strong enough
19. I am grateful / appreciative	19. I am different
20. I am an uplifter	20. I am selfish

Let's just take a look at a few examples. Take a look at how many of my **Fear** insights on the rights and see how they COMPLETELY CONTRADICTED my **Love** insights on the left!

LIFE MILESTONES: Love or Fear The Contradictions Corner	
LOVE	**FEAR**
LOVE #1 - I am strong	FEAR #18 - I am not strong enough
LOVE #4 - I am smart	FEAR #2 - I am not smart enough
LOVE #7 - I am not a quitter	FEAR #13 - I am afraid to fail
LOVE #9 - I am courageous	FEAR #4 - I am fearful
LOVE #11 - I create big goals for myself	FEAR #9 - I am not confident
LOVE #15 - I am an inspirer	FEAR#5 - I am full of self-doubt

Like what??? Who are these two people living in my body? How did these two separate exercises yield such crazy contradictions? Why do we judge ourselves so harshly on our failures, when we know when we look through the lens of love, that we are strong, brave, talented and connected to our source, our true spirit?

It is a lens of duality my friends. We all have it. Ying and Yang. Positive and Negative. But it is the thing that stops us and limits our thoughts, decisions and aspirations. We need only to look at our list of love...which is our truth.

Let's do yours.

Take a moment and compare your lists. Do you find equal contradictions between your love and fear self?

LIFE MILESTONES: Love or Fear The Contradictions Corner	
LOVE	**FEAR**

Take a few minutes to dig deep into these contradictions and what the meaning behind this message may be for your soul. Again, this would be a great place for you to write a few thoughts on your 'aha's' that come to you as a result of doing this exercise. Which column do you really believe?

Dying to Be Ourselves

Taking these important steps to explore how our deeply embedded beliefs of love and fear, infiltrate and influence our belief system, can literally change the course of our lives. I'd like to end this chapter with the story of a woman who was near death, within her last moments of life, able to see the light and beauty of her soul for the very first time.

On February 2, 2006 after fighting cancer for almost four years, Anita Moorjani fell into a coma and was given hours to live. As her body and organs shut down, Anita journeyed into a near-death experience (NDE) in which she says she was surrounded by "unconditional love and deep wisdom." In this expanded state, she was able to see herself and her life experience with the enlightened clarity of unconditional love. Anita felt completely bathed and renewed in this energy, as though she finally belonged. In her words, she had finally "come home."

Anita was given the choice to return to her body or stay in this expansive new realm. After deep reflection, she chose to come back. When she awoke, to the amazement of her doctors, her health immediately began to improve and she was cancer-free within weeks. She went from literally being within hours of death, to a complete recovery, that despite the amazement of her doctors, defied a scientific explanation.

Anita went on to write the New York Times bestseller, *Dying to Be Me*, sharing her profoundly inspiring story of how this renewed understanding of her soul's purpose brought her quite literally back to life.

> "I instinctively understood that I was dying because of all my fears," Anita wrote. In that expansive state, I realized how harshly I'd treated myself and judged myself throughout my life... I was the one who was judging me, whom I'd forsaken, and whom I didn't love enough…. I saw that I'd never loved myself, valued myself, or seen the beauty of my own soul."

It was with renewed understanding of her purpose that Anita finally understood how she carried the weight and judgement of herself from a place of fear, and that so much of her life was lived on the pretense of making everyone else happy at her own expense.

> "As I looked at the great tapestry that was the accu-mulation of my life up to that point, I was able to identify exactly what had brought me to where I was today. Just look at my life path! Why, oh why, have I always been so harsh with myself? Why was I always beating myself up? Why was I always for-saking myself? Why did I never stand up for myself and show the world the beauty of my own soul? Why was I always suppressing my own intelligence and creativity to please others? I betrayed myself every time I said yes when I meant no! Why have I violated myself by always needing to seek approval from

others just to be myself? Why haven't I followed my own beautiful heart and spoken my own truth? Why don't we realize this when we're in our physical bodies? How come I never knew that we're not supposed to be so tough on ourselves? I still felt myself completely enveloped in a sea of unconditional love and acceptance. I was able to look at myself with fresh eyes, and I saw that I was a beautiful being of the Universe."

According to Anita, her work, in this lifetime, is to show others what she has come to learn herself. To let go of the worry, the doubt and the negative self-talk, the toxic emotions that eventually caused the "dis-ease" which she believes ultimately became the cancer that overtook her body. In her words, it just came down to that magical but oh so difficult choice between love and fear. "I just had to be myself, fearlessly!" she wrote. "In that way, I'd be allowing myself to be an instrument of love. I understood that this was the best thing that any of us could possibly do or be, for both the planet and ourselves."

Anita would go on to write another book and travel the world sharing her message that everything that happens in our lives has a potentially positive meaning for us…even the most difficult experiences. "Everything that seemingly happens externally is occurring in order to trigger something within us," she wrote "Your only work is to love yourself, value yourself, and embody this truth of self-worth and self-love so that you can be love in action. That is true service, to yourself and to those who surround you."

It's as if Anita has already created her own LifeMap!

Sometimes, when the seemingly worst things happen to us, we don't understand the "power" we have over our reaction to the situation. It can be easy to blame God, the circumstances or other people. We can decide that there is no hope, or that we are the victim of a specific outcome. But no matter what the situation is, I promise you, the choice is always ours.

Your biggest life challenge, your most incomprehensible fear, can be THE very thing that shows you your purpose – what you have come into this world to do. When you are most afraid, close your eyes and focus only on love…let it fill you and surround you. There you will find the heart of your soul, your endless resource of power and strength.

You are braver and more powerful than you know!

In the next chapter, you'll see how your beautiful milestones intertwine with your soul mates and guides, weaving together still another magical layer of your wonderful life's tapestry.

Be inspired. Like Santiago, you have already come far on your own hero's journey. You are following your own north star.

> "The boy rode along through the desert…listening avidly to what his heart had to say. 'Where your treasure is, there will be your heart,' the alchemist had told him…As he was about to climb yet another dune, his heart whispered, "Be aware of the place where you are brought to tears. That's where I am, and that's where your treasure is."
>
> (The Alchemist p.164)

SOUL GOODY BAG

Here are some resources mentioned in this chapter for you for further exploration:

- **The Alchemist by Paulo Coelho** tells the magical story of Santiago, a shepherd boy who travels the world in search of treasure. Santiago's journey shares the essential wisdom of listening to our hearts, learning to read the signs along life's path and, above all, following our dreams.

- **Dying to Be Me by Anita Moorgani**-In *Dying to Be Me*, Anita freely shares all she has learned about illness, healing, fear, "being love," and the true magnificence of each and every human being! This is a book that definitely makes the case that we are spiritual beings having a human experience . . . and that we are all One!

- **KatherineofLight** – For more information on Light language...contact Katherine on her Facebook page at katherineoflight.

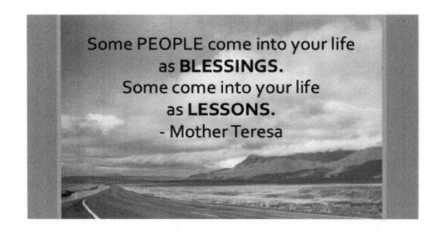

Some PEOPLE come into your life
as **BLESSINGS.**
Some come into your life
as **LESSONS.**
- Mother Teresa

CHAPTER 7

LESSONS FROM YOUR SQUAD

"How we find and recognize our soul mates and the life-transforming decisions we must then make, are among the most moving and important decisions in our lives. Destiny dictates the meeting of soul mates. We *will* meet them. But what we decide to do after that meeting, falls in the province of choice or free will."

These words launch the first chapter of "Only Love is Real," written by New York Times best- selling author, Dr. Brian Weiss. The book is about soul mates...people in Weiss's words "who are bonded eternally by their love and who come around together again and again, life after life." The publication was written as a follow up to his earlier revolutionary book "Many Lives, Many Masters," in which Weiss shares his accidental discovery and documentation of multiple past life memories that surfaces during sessions with one of his patients.

His work inspired millions as he put both science and curiosity behind his work, inspiring millions about this loving, timeless connection to our loved ones. "You may be awakened to the presence of your soul companion by a look, a dream, a memory, a feeling..." Weiss writes. "The touch that awakens may be that of your child, a parent, a sibling or of a true friend. Or it may be your beloved, reaching across centuries, to kiss you once again and to remind you that you are together always, to the end of time."

I mean...how does real love get better than that?

Welcome to "Lessons from your Squad!"– we have so much to talk about!!

In this chapter, we'll explore some of the specific lessons we are offered from our soul mates, these amazing members of our divine family who have chosen to incarnate with us to romp, wander and kick up the dirt of earth with us. This delightful group have chosen to take the journey for the love they have for us...just without the memory of "why" we came together. Is that not a definition of brave, selfless love?

In this chapter, we will cut through our earthly amnesia and identify what the key people in your life have already taught you about yourself, and the HOW that's impacted your life's path. Here's our plan for this last plot through the past.

- **Soul Mate Examples** - I will share a few deeply personal stories about how I faced my own darkest fears with the help of two key members of my soul squad, who have taught me and the rest of my soul family incredible lessons of love, courage and forgiveness. Without an understanding of eternal connection, our earthly circumstances could have crushed our spirits with despair, blame and isolation.

- **Soul Mate Categories** -Your vision of a true soul mate may be tainted by movies and fairy tales. Real soul mates have different faces and roles, and they are not always the romantic kind.
- **Soul Mapping Your Mates**-We'll follow the same exercise as we did with our milestones, to reveal some of the amazing lessons your Squad has already offered you.
- **Bless and Release** –We'll finish this section with a powerful offering to our squad sending love and releasing anything from the past that will keep us attached to any fear-based memories that no longer serves us.

So, let's jump in, shall we? I'll share stories about two of my most powerful soul mates and teachers, Graham and Cyndi. I love them both so much for offering significant parts of their lives to teach me the meaning of love. I hope their stories will inspire you to think about some of your own experiences through a different lens and recognize the beautiful soul mates who might be living under your own roof or close around you.

First, I will share Graham's story. He has taught me every-thing about living and loving fiercely, and how a toddler (with a little family help) was able to perform miracles.

My Littlest Teacher – The Story of Graham.

The automatic doors of the hospital sprang open like a mechanical hand snatching us from our everyday lives, casting us into the vast, controlled chaos of the ER. It was January 18, 2001, and inside those doors, there was no turning back.

We pulled off our jackets and grabbed the last remaining chairs in the waiting room. My husband, Ralph, approached the admission desk. When the receptionist asked if we had been there before, Ralph nodded; our son Graham's information had already become a fixture in their database.

Seven months before, Graham had been born in this hospital. With joyful relief, we had welcomed him into our arms, swaddled his healthy, hearty, little body with love and gave thanks. With tearful relief, I watched Ralph, with his heart and arms full of newfound fatherhood, follow the nurse down the hallway to his son's first bath...

And that's the last thing I remembered that day.

"We need you to come back Karen...squeeze my hand if you can hear me." Somewhere far away, I heard Ralph's voice. My body felt too heavy to move but his urgency pulled me out of my grogginess. When I opened my eyes, I saw my tearful husband standing over me. When I tried to speak, my voice caught in my throat.

"You're on a breathing tube honey...try not to talk."

I was confused...what was I doing there? My last memory was of giving birth to my son. The joy of seeing his beautiful face... 'oh God,' I panicked, 'where was my baby?'

As if reading my mind, Ralph said, "The baby is fine, Karen. He's with your Mom downstairs. You're in the ICU. You've been here for days...you gave us all quite a scare."

After the delivery I had a hemorrhage and ended up with emergency surgery and a series of blood transfusions that saved my life. For days afterwards, I was in an induced coma, saved I am certain by the deep love of my husband and family, as well as a steady stream of Reiki healers, arranged by my vigilant Mother, who worked on me while I slept. I remembered thinking, "that's the closest I EVER want to get to a near-death experience, ever again."

Thankfully, I recovered quickly, and we went home days later, returning to a new family "normal". Graham quickly grew into a precocious ball of smiles. Healthy, happy, thriving...

Until he wasn't.

In early November, our babysitter called me at work. "Karen, Graham has been throwing up again. I think he should get looked at by the doctor." We had been alternating from breast milk to formula and a new regime of food, which seemed to have triggered an ongoing series of stomach issues.

The Pediatrician affirmed that his new diet was the culprit. He suggested some alternatives but, three weeks later, we were back with similar symptoms, only Graham had a fever this time. In my mind, I heard the siren of a mother's instinct bellow a loud cry of warning. But for what?

Graham continued to yoyo between seemingly normal health and bouts of vomiting. In early January, I'd planned a surprise 40th birthday party for Ralph and my Mom came to help. She hadn't seen Graham in a few weeks and pulled me aside. "Karen, you have to get him to another doctor. When did he get that bump on his head?"

What bump? Suddenly, I saw the small lump on his forehead and was terrified. We immediately went to the ER.

As we waited, Grahams fever climbed. He was listless and dehydrated. During the examination, the doctor noticed his rigid belly and said that the bump on his head could be symptomatic of a few causes, including a brain tumor. He ordered a spinal tap and CAT Scan. We waited in agony for the results.

Graham was diagnosed with stage four neuroblastoma; a one in a million cancer, that primarily affects very young children. The cancer had spread to his bones, including his skull, causing the bump on his head and he had a tumor the size of a lemon in his adrenal gland. He needed immediate surgery to remove the tumor, followed by rounds of in-patient chemotherapy. We were scheduled to meet with a team of pediatric oncologists immediately.

What followed was my lowest point as a mother.

As the doctor continued his diagnosis, I held Graham's limp, sleeping body in my arms and went inwardly numb. I felt the fear sear like lightning bolts through my veins. Like that moment in the ICU, when my voice was caught in my throat. An inward scream of "I CAN'T do this!" slashed through my heart. I placed Graham in his father's arms and said, "My son is going to die," and ran out of the room.

My mother followed me down the hall. "Karen, this is an unbelievable situation. We're all scared but Graham needs you and I know you can do this. You CAN."

Behind her was her ever-resilient daughter, Lauren, and my strong, courageous husband who held our son and said, "Karen, we are going to get through this. We will do this together. He is going to be fine."

I looked at my little boy who still managed to smile through his pain and sickness, then stretched his little arms back to me for a hug of reassurance. "Okay", I said, "Let's do this."

The following weeks of treatment were a blur. Of cradling his weak head while nurses ran an IV from his skull because he was so dehydrated that they couldn't find a vein. Of placing his tiny body on the operating table and leaving him in the hands of masked strangers. Of waiting for news on how each round of chemo was impacting the prognosis of recovery or...not.

Numerous moments tested our faith in the months that followed. White cell counts that were too low or too high. Fevers that spiked in the middle of the night requiring late night ambulance rides to the ER. But we became a strong family unit. We got good at keeping charts, and check-in lists, and action plans. Of being the watchdog and protector of anything and anyone that touched our child. We questioned the so-called medical authorities and double checked every prescription script and diagnosis. We lived in the moment. We prayed all the time. We slept in increments. But we never spoke of the possibility of Graham dying ever again.

And that was how we took our power back.

This was a defining moment for us because it gave us the strength to choose love over fear.

And in doing so...hope and openness and possibility became our mantras. We learned to trust in things seen and unseen. We opened to alternative medicines and holistic modalities to enhance Graham's recovery outside of conventional medicine. We learned about energy healing and positive thinking. We looked for angels everywhere. We visualized and affirmed that Graham was well. We opened our hearts and minds to the kindness of strangers. We learned to live in the moment; truly the toughest lesson for two madly controlling corporate parents who wanted to use our management skills to create the project plan around our child's recovery. Graham reminded us to play. We savored every moment. Our family unit reigned. We were a force of love to be reckoned with.

And Graham got well.

I received a card during Graham's illness that had a quote from the great writer Marianne Williamson that said, "*A miracle is a shift in perception from fear to love.*" Inside the card, was another quote, "*If you knew who walked beside you at all times, you would never experience fear or doubt ever again. Where there is great love, there are always miracles.*" I re-read those words often. They came true for us.

Graham recently graduated from high school. He doesn't remember a lot about those trips to the hospital, but we share the stories and the photos with him every year on his cancer-free birthday which ironically happens every September 11th. He will always be a living, breathing miracle for us.

Today, we live on the other side of the dark tunnel and share our story with other parents who have and are still facing their fears with all the courage they can muster. We tell them to hold on tight and keep their eyes on the light. We tell them that it is love that will get them through the fear.

From Coward to Courageous

I share this story with you because this experience has been one of my most powerful teachers. It was a life lesson that was orchestrated with my soul mates....my husband, my son, my daughter, my mother and family...the doctors and nurses, were all part of this amazing co-creative experience with the center of the stage, Graham. In it I see both my strength and my weakness...where I've been both a coward, and courageous.

As I said before, sometimes when the seemingly worst things happen to us, we don't understand the "power" we ourselves have over our reaction to the situation. We maybe tempted to blame God, the circumstances or other people. We can decide that there is no hope, or that we are the victim of fate. Or we can decide that we can see past the facts, to a vision of the possible. Or in our case, to an affirmation like...*the diagnosis is not the prognosis*.

Because no matter what the situation is, I promise you, **it's always up to us to choose what we believe.**

There is no doubt that Graham, Ralph and Lauren, my parents and our many friends who walked beside us during this harrowing journey from death back to health are part of my soul squad – a magical band of life learners who have come together in this life to help us love Graham back to life and to create a miracle.

"A miracle" according to Marianne Williamson, "is a shift in perception from fear to love." Think about the power of that!

If you too are facing a journey into the dark night of your soul, I urge you to look for those who can be part of your soul squad. They can be family or friend, animal or angel, living with us on the planet or beside us on the other side. Never forget that no one is here on this journey completely alone. We have all come here with teachers who are hand in hand, shoulder to shoulder, and heart to heart...part of our team to help show us the way.

In the beautiful words of Dr. Brian Weiss "When allowed to flow freely, love overcomes all obstacles."

Carrying our Connections from Lifetime to Lifetime: Exploring Past Lives

So how can I have so much certainty about the squad? These so-called teachers and love enablers who have joined us on our soul journey? Well, I have proof of course!

You see, as it turns out, there are trained intuitive counselors who can help us tap into remembering our soul lessons and why we chose to come back to hang through this lifetime together.

Years after Graham's cancer experience, I had the opportunity to meet with the incredible Michelle Brock, a New York City based spiritual development life coach, who specializes in past life regression.

In my case, I was there out of my fascination with the process, and curiosity (and a little fear) about what my session would uncover. Michelle was trained by Dr. Brian Weiss, and integrates, a carefully guided meditation, visualization and intuition, which invites the memories of our past life experiences to resurface.

With Michelle's expert guidance, I was able to reconnect with two of my prior lifetimes. In the first memory, I recalled a lifetime that appeared to take place in the 1500's in Scotland. I was getting ready to attend a large social gathering of some kind, and was getting ready in a large room that looked like it was in a castle or large estate. Outside, I could see my father (the same father as I have in this lifetime) standing next to a horse drawn carriage below my window. I knew he was still grieving the passing of my mother (who was my maternal grandmother in this lifetime) who had recently died from a long illness. I knew it was my father's hope that I would find a suitor at the event so I could be safely married and live a secure life with a husband. I wasn't excited about the prospect of moving on.

As I walked through the crowd in the great hall, there was a long row of knights standing on either side of the walkway...that I understood were the young suitors who were lined up for the dance. I scanned the group, with a sigh of boredom, and then....one familiar face caught my eye....it was Ralph, looking back at me with a twinkle of recognition in his eyes! Well, I'll be darned I thought...that's why I am here. I laughed out loud recalling my pleased irony in that moment...it was a memory that was real!

Michelle then had me fast forward from that event to a later part of that same lifetime. I could see that I had just given birth to a baby boy...my son Graham. My daughter Lauren was also there. I could see their faces...in the dark candle-lit room. The baby was fine...but I wasn't...there was sadness ... I could feel myself drifting away and I died.

The incredible emotion that accompanied this memory was like nothing else I've ever experienced. The depth of sadness of leaving my family behind... of feeling their loneliness without me...of knowing that it was just the three of them and how my death left such a hole in their lives. Their grief as real as my own.

With Michelle's help, I was able to release some of that deep sadness and regret...as well a realization of how recalling that experience had a message for my current life. It helped me understand the depth of my family's need for me to "be there" and the important role I play in "centering" our family connection. It also provided insight on how, because of my work obligations, my family is "used to" the fact that I am not there, but there is still a feeling of emptiness when I'm gone.

This experience helped me see the many dimensions and dynamics of my present families' relationship, and that I have signed up to "repeat" my learnings with them again because we were not able to complete our experience in our last life together. This is another round for closeness, communication, time, attention, and family love that we lost in the last one.

Ok, just a couple of notes to share on this.

If you have not had an opportunity for a past life session with a truly gifted regressionist like Michelle, I realize that this might be a hard experience to imagine. I had so many friends respond with both interest and skeptics that these hypnotic recollections had to be made up or induced by our imagination. But here's the one universal takeaway that I believe is the way to benchmark the truth of the experience for yourself- you **FEEL the emotion** attached to memory. You cry, you feel longing, fear and familiarity. There is a full feeling with that memory which would not be attached to something your mind has just imagined. And the other piece? You **DON'T FORGET the emotion**, the visual certainty of what you saw...it stays with you.

Past life regression is an incredible tool to further connect and clarify the purpose of your current lifetime. Since only our bodies die but our souls live on, we hold so many of our memories and lessons deep within our spiritual knowing, from lifetime to lifetime. Michelle explained that very often, people utilize past life regression therapy as a way of uncovering reasons why they may have certain unexplained phobias, anxieties or are just struggling with difficult relationships with family members. It's all an ongoing part of our growth that we carry with us always.

Take a moment and think about this in your own life. Is it possible that you can find situations or people that could potentially be part of your soul pod that are with you in this life? When you see your son, or sibling, do you see an old soul looking back at you?

Since our session, Michelle shared with me some insights into her own Seeker's journey that helped her understand her life's mission to help others connect to their past in order to heal. Like my medium friend, Lisa Nitzkin, Michelle also lost her mother at a very young age, but found that the subsequent death of her grandmother triggered her understanding of her life's purpose. It was through her grief and reaching for meaning that she was able to reconnect with her mother and spirit guides who were willing soul mates ready to help teach her from the other side.

Seeker Stories:

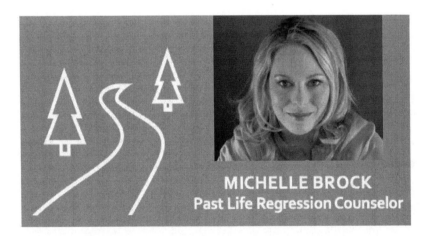

MICHELLE BROCK
Past Life Regression Counselor

The most pivotal moment of my life came right after I had experienced an incredible spiritual awakening. My grandmother, whom I adored, had just died. Losing her brought back the feelings of losing my mother all over again, even though she had died 30 years prior.

I was in a marriage that was literally hanging by a thread and had two babies under the age of 2. And, on top of this, we had just moved away from all of my family and friends to a different state for my husband's job. He was always busy and away, leaving me to care for a toddler and an infant completely on my own. I had never felt so alone.

Around this time, I was given the book, "Many Lives, Many Masters," by Dr. Brian Weiss, that lead me on a journey to discover myself on a deep, soul level. This book, which introduced the idea that I had lived before in a past life, uncovered actual memories from my own past lives. This changed the way that I looked at everything. This insight opened new eyes for me on spiritual concepts that I had never even contemplated. However, the most important shift from this profound spiritual awakening was that the circumstances of my life reflected my own choices. That insight, that my feelings of being lonely and dis-connected from others didn't need to be true, meant that I had to take responsibility for my own life and my own happiness.

Once I had discovered that past lives were real, that also meant that soul mates were real as well. And that there were others who were journeying alongside me over many lifetimes, soul mates that I had reconnected with already and soul mates that were still waiting to be found. I just had to change the way that I looked at these connections and choose to have deep, spiritual, soul mate connections with the people in my life. I knew that I had to take the incredible spiritual experience I had as a sign that there was more for me to explore. I knew this meant that I should aspire to have a deeper, spiritual love with the soul mates in my life.

Since that pivotal moment when I realized that I had to change how I was living, how I looked at my life, and push past the fear and doubt that kept me from fully embracing the beliefs that were created by this unique spiritual experience. The truth was, I needed to choose how much love I created in my life and how much love I allowed myself to receive. And now I am surrounded by love and I never feel alone, as I have so many soul mates of many different types. I am truly blessed.

Our Soul Squad Connections

Like Michelle, I love the lessons offered in past life regression because I am so certain that we all have intricate, multi-dimensional, pre-life contracts with each other. Every person who comes into our lives is our teacher. It is up to us to see the lessons.

As we continue our life mapping, identifying the key people in our lives will help us understand this magical inter-woven tapestry of connection.

Identifying the Roles of Our Squad:

In Chapter Four, we learned *How to Recognize the people in our soul team.*

We learned there are "**Teachers,**" like our parents and partners, who are here to help us learn very specific life lessons about love and fear. They tend to be the ones who have the most long-term impact on our root beliefs about ourselves and the world. There are also "**Triggers**" and "**Kindreds**" who offer us opportunities that help us develop and evaluate our own instincts and preferences. And then there the "**Disrupters**" and the "**Connectors**" who tend to enter and exit through our lives like human bumper cars, sometimes causing us to veer off course, or head down a new or completely unexpected path.

In our next Lifemapping exercise, we'll look at the very specific roles these souls have had in your life. Regardless of the amount of "time" they may have interacted with you, this will really help you understand what you have "signed up for" to experience together.

Here are the **Four Soul Mate Categories**:

1. **Family** – You came together to experience inter-action as a "unit" or "relative"– to test the bonds and beliefs of a human family or group united not necessarily by preference, but by birth or marriage, carrying with it genetic and ancestorial messages, beliefs, and expectations. These are your elders and your descendants…your parents and grandparents, your children, your spouses, your in-laws, and your stepfamilies. The layer on which you build on…your roots, your soul's DNA…**They are part of your life's "foundation."**

2. **Friend** – You come together in mutual recognition of each other. You complement each other's talents, interests, hobbies, careers, personalities. Your friend recognizes the real you without judgement…not for who you are married to, the home you live in, the car that you drive, the career you do or don't have. They have your best interests at heart. **They are your "support system"** who softly surrounds your life with no strings attached.

3. **Influencer** – You came together around an idea, emotion or feeling that leaves an impression within you. This is someone who tells you a story, introduces you to a political idea or belief, who offers you an opportunity to grow or make a difference. This person MOVES you. While you don't experience the level of intimacy that you might with a romantic love or friend, they impact you in a unique way, that changes you. **They are your "aspirational source"** offering you to do, be or believe in something.

4. **Partner** - You came together in a pairing with another that "sees" you, heart to heart. They rivet your mind, body and spirit, and inspire your highest levels of emotion, passion, as well as self and mutual love. There is a level of intimacy and connection that goes beyond the physical, as if there is an invisible chord of light that connects you soul to soul. **They are the connection to "your inspiration"** to your spirit or your "higher self," because they cause you to desire...within as well as with out, to help us see and remember our full, true spirit, which is love.

If you are reading through this now, and are being tripped up on the "romance" part of love or if you feel you have not found that in your life yet, I would add that soul mates, do not necessarily have to be physical human beings. All of the ideas above can also be "a place," or even a thing or an object. Faith or Religion can be part of your foundational soul "family." A pet or animal could serve as part of your support system and the best possible "friend." A life-changing "influencer" could be a song, or a musical instrument, or a hobby that aspires a thought, feeling or desire within you. And you could have a long and fulfilling "romance" with a city, or a house that you live in, because it instills a passionate feeling of love and inspiration within you. You need not have a relationship with a person to create a life fulling experience but the people who come into your life that provide you with these meaningful human interactions, do so as your soul mates.

Dr. Brian Weiss added context to this. In "Only Love is Real," he says, "You may not always marry your most strongly bonded soulmate. There may be more than one for you, because would families travel together, your strongest soulmate connection may be to your parent, or to your child, or to your sibling. Or your strongest connection may be to a soulmate who has not incarnated during your lifetime and who is watching over you from the other side, like a guardian angel.

As you go through your life map milestones, you may also find that some of the above roles may overlap or meld into each other. A good friend who became a romantic partner, or a relative may become your greatest influencer. These are your soul mates who are paramount forces in your life, and have the most impact on you. Keep note of the intensity of how the pendulum swings emotionally with these relationships as these will show you some of the key experiences you have come to learn.

Curious what this all means for you? Let us carry on!

Setting Your Intention

Again, we have another wonderful opportunity to pause and give thanks to those wonderful beings who have joined us on this wild adventure we call life. And whatever the lesson they have brought with them for us, we have the chance today to remember that we always have the power to choose the influence that they have had on us. We decide how any given experience will impact our lives from this point forward.

SOULFIRMATION #7

"Today I set my intention to see my soul mates as they truly are...
We are co-creators...
Playmates in this limitless sandbox of life
And as we build and reshape together,
We know that our time is both temporary and infinite.
That our physical walk is but a moment in our forever eternity
That our being in human form is just our spirits expanding and evolving.
We thank each and every mate who has offered us such love to journey with our soul
To be with us in our forgetfulness...until we leave our masks behind and reunite with truth again".

EXERCISE: Take a deep breath in...imagine your breath is love. Hold it in as long as you can. Visualize your breath, swirling around inside your lungs and solar plexus...becoming infused with a pastel color of pink that is warmed by the love in your heart.

And as you exhale, imagine your breath.... now a beautiful pink color, leaving your body and going out to the world... off to those wonderful soul guides and mates that have touched your life in some way.

Repeat as often as you like, directing your heart infused breaths surrounding and becoming the breath of those wonderful beings who have been part of you, your foundation, your support system, your aspirations and inspirations.

See they know you are sending them this love and how it, in turn, loves them from the inside out. I do this exercise whenever I want to send peace, or thanks, or support or forgiveness to my mates.

You can do it when you are driving, or out for a run, or in the shower, or as you are falling asleep.

It is powerful... and it will fill you with light.

LIFEMAPPING EXPLORATION #6

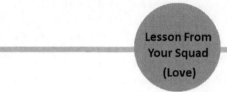

In the last chapter when we decoded our Love and Fear Milestones, we were able to take a look at how each of them played a role in how we felt about our lives. We were able to really look at the meaning and impact of each encounter and create "I am" belief statements that were associated with each experience.

Now we are going to take a look at our soul mates in the same way. And we will follow the same steps as we did in our prior exercise. So again, because we are going back in time, we need to be mindful of our energy in taking the journey to revisit both these happy and difficult moments.

So, the same guidelines apply.

Lifemapping Reminder: Before we start, a reminder of our grounding rules.

1. Give yourself a time limit – 15 minutes is a good goal for this exploration.
2. As in our prior exercises, find a comfortable location for you to do this work.
3. Try not to overthink it.
4. Be gentle with yourself – if this becomes too emotional for one sitting, you can divide this exercise into parts, or come back when you are ready.

Part One: The "I AM" Lessons from our "Love Mates"

As we did before, we are going to center our first exercise on LOVE…. but rather than looking at the experiences themselves, we are focusing on the people who were the life-shapers on our journey.

Here is the process to follow:

Step 1: Identify Go back to the list of the soul mates who you listed in your Lifemapping exercise in Chapter 4 who were part of the love moments in your life. In each circle on the outside of your list, add their name.

Step 2: Evaluate – Picture that person in your mind again. Relive some of those memories with them. How did this person make you feel?

Step 3: Actualize – Write the "I am" statement that translates what that person taught you about your own worthiness. You can write more than one "I am" statement per person if there were multiple lessons learned from this person.

Step 4: Reflect - When you have completed your list, take an few extra minutes to capture in your journal how these "I am" statements feel for you.

- Do they surprise you?
- Do they help you remember anything about yourself that you might have forgotten?
- Do you believe them?

You may be tempted to go back and look at how some of your "I am" statements that you wrote in our Decoding

Exercise in the last chapter, compare to the ones you write about your soul mates here. But I would encourage you to hold on to that for now, as we will use this information in another exploration that is coming up soon.

As a reference, you will also see my own Lifemapping exercise here…just in case you want some ideas.

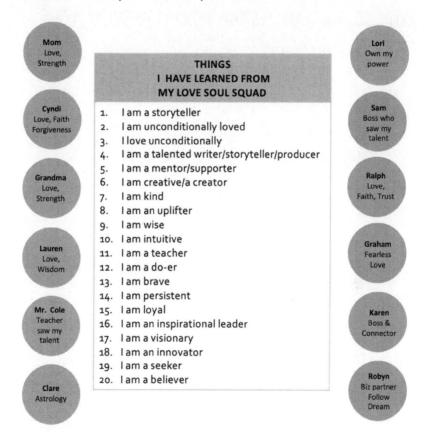

Mom Love, Strength

Cyndi Love, Faith Forgiveness

Grandma Love, Strength

Lauren Love, Wisdom

Mr. Cole Teacher saw my talent

Clare Astrology

Lori Own my power

Sam Boss who saw my talent

Ralph Love, Faith, Trust

Graham Fearless Love

Karen Boss & Connector

Robyn Biz partner Follow Dream

THINGS
I HAVE LEARNED FROM
MY LOVE SOUL SQUAD

1. I am a storyteller
2. I am unconditionally loved
3. I love unconditionally
4. I am a talented writer/storyteller/producer
5. I am a mentor/supporter
6. I am creative/a creator
7. I am kind
8. I am an uplifter
9. I am wise
10. I am intuitive
11. I am a teacher
12. I am a do-er
13. I am brave
14. I am persistent
15. I am loyal
16. I am an inspirational leader
17. I am a visionary
18. I am an innovator
19. I am a seeker
20. I am a believer

To do this, I chose my biggest soul squad leaders, jotted a thought or two within the circle about their role, and then created my "I am statements" describing how they taught me about love and myself around those lessons.

So much to learn, know and understand and it is all creating the beautiful vision that is you.

OK – you have the plan for the exercise and the template is on the next page.

Go with LOVE!

EXERCISE: THE "I AM "LESSONS FROM YOUR SQUAD: LOVE

- **Step 1: Identify** -The soul mates who were part of the love moments in your life. Add their name to the circle.

- **Step 2: Evaluate** - Relive some of those memories. How did this person make you feel?

- **Step 3: Actualize** - Write the "I am" statement that translates what that person taught you about your own worthiness.

- **Step 4: Reflect** - When you have completed your list, take an few extra minutes to capture in your journal how these "I am" statement feel for you.

THINGS I HAVE LEARNED FROM MY LOVE SOUL SQUAD
1.
2.
3.
4.
5.
6.
7.
8.
9.
10.
11.
12.
13.
14.
15.
16.
17.
18.
19.
20.

Lessons from My Lifemap: My Soul Squad/Love Connection Milestones

When I did this exercise for the first time, it filled me with so much gratitude! I had so many wonderful people come in and out of my life, and it felt so good to take some time to truly appreciate all of the "LOVE" that had been offered to me in this lifetime.

My Mom and Grandmother, my dearest girlfriends, my high school writing teacher, a few of my bosses and mentors, my amazing daughter, and my giving husband. I was so blessed to have these dear loving soul mates as part of my tribe. I have found that my best teachers have been and continue to be the ones who have been able to truly see the real, authentic me...the ones where I was able to shine the inner light that was me...and they RECOGNIZED me.

Is that how you felt too? Do you remember that feeling of "oh my gosh...they SEE me! And the love the me that is me???!!! It is joy...It is this feeling of exuberant, blissful...relief!

That you can expose yourself in all of your naked truthfulness...and you are appreciated for all that you really are...not what you pretend to be. They are true soul mates and teachers who recognize the essence of our hearts who help amplify the good within us.

When I look back at my life's biggest milestones, it was clear that my soul squad was really there at the times when I needed them most. Filling out my circles and writing my LOVE "I am " affirmations came fairly easily. They made me feel proud, accomplished and valued. And putting my takeaways from those milestones created a feeling like I was in fact living on purpose.

Finding our Soul Tribe through Grief

As we saw in Katherine's story in the last chapter, and Michelle's story earlier in this one, some of our biggest life milestones can come through heartbreak. Failed marriages and severed family relationships/friendships can mean both physical and emotional deaths that can shatter the very foundations of who we are. Consequently, this can call in to question the meaning of everything we hold true.

In this next story, you will hear from my Mom and personal hero, and fellow Lifemapper, Lo Anne Mayer, on how she was able to face the biggest fear of all: Death. Through unimaginable tragedy and loss, Lo Anne was able to find her way back to the light and, with the help of her mother and daughter soul mates, she offers her story of healing and hope helping thousands around the world heal through their grief.

LOANNE'S STORY: How Grief Rewrote A Mothers Story

Lo Anne raised her six children in the New Jersey suburbs. She was a devoted mother with a strong faith, and spent her life dedicated to caring for her family. With her children grown and off on their own life's adventures, she was embarking on her own mid-life quest as a spiritual seeker, teacher, Reiki master and writer.

In July 2005, Lo Anne was invited to join a group of friends and travel to Glastonbury, England for a weeklong writer's conference. At first, she hesitated to make the trip. Her daughter Cyndi was going through a bitter divorce that included a custody battle over her two grandsons, one of whom was autistic.

But with her husband's encouragement, Lo Anne decided to take the trip, and was quickly mesmerized by the beautiful Abby House in Glastonbury; a magical retreat center in the cemetery ruins where it was said that King Arthur was buried. In her words, "Glastonbury seemed to be a doorway between the worlds of fact and imagination, heaven and earth, life and death."

On the fourth day of the conference, Lo Anne was called to the hotel's front desk for a phone call. She slumped to the ground in shock as her husband broke the news that Cyndi had committed suicide.

Despite her strong faith and belief in the afterlife, Lo Anne could not process what had happened, and the pain of being so far away at the time of her daughter's passing. There were so many details that she couldn't piece together. What was going through Cyndi's mind that drove her to such an extreme choice? Did she suffer and feel abandoned when she died? Was she really ok and being taken care of by the angels on the other side? Suddenly, all of Lo Anne's own teachings were in question. Her pre-conceived certainty of the afterlife shattered to its core.

As she prepared for the wake and funeral of her daughter, Lo Anne did the only thing she could think of. She wrote a letter to her dead mother.

In the years prior to Cyndi's death, Lo Anne had utilized a practice she called "transpersonal journaling" to communicate with her own Mother after she died. Grieving over the strained relationship they endured in life and longing for healing, Lo Anne had started a collaborative journal – a dialogue of "celestial conversations" between her and her mother. In the writing, they were able to "correspond" and share soul-to-soul communications that restored their bond.

Overwhelmed with grief, Lo Anne sought her mother's help in how to cope with the loss of her daughter. "*Mother, I need help.*" Lo Anne wrote in the early morning hours before Cyndi's service. "*I need to know from you that Cyndi is alright. I need to know that you are together. I need your help in processing the unfathomable...*"

The next day, a response came from her mother with an answered prayer and a surprise.

"*Dear Lo Anne- I am here with Cyndi. She is fine...I am here helping her process...loving her and loving you.*"

"We are with you, Cyndi and I," her mother added *"...we surround you with our love and healing... Choose the forgiveness road no matter what your mind tells you. There is no other way..."*

Suddenly, the tone and penmanship of the message changed. *"Mom, I am so sorry to cause you and Daddy so much pain..."* Cyndi words came through in her journal...it was as if she could hear her voice. *"I am so very sorry."* This was the beginning of a new trans-journaling communication that Lo Anne would continue with her daughter from the other side that would help heal them both.

In the weeks and months that followed, Lo Anne continued the trans-journaling process with her mother and daughter. Five years later, Lo Anne's book, that she wrote in partnership with her mother and daughter, "Celestial Conversations, Healing Relationships After Death," was published. From that point on, Lo Anne and her husband Ray began sharing the book and their story with thousands of grieving people around the world.

My Soul Tribe Circle of Grief

Lo Anne's story is my mother's story. It is my sister's story. It is my family's story. It is my story. We have all been part of this soul journey together. When my sister left the planet, we all stepped into a role that none of us ever wanted. The Soul Tribe Circle of Grief.

While my mom was attending her writing class in Glastonbury, I also happened to be flying to London the same week to produce a video project for AT&T. We had joked as we were prepping for our mutual trips that it would be fun if we could make time for us to meet up while we were there, as the last time we were in the UK together was when I was attending Oxford University as a college student. "It's a sign Mom," I said, "Maybe we could meet there for a little walk down memory lane."

As it turned out, the synchronicity of our journey's would be far more important than we realized. I was shooting the last segment of our show under the London Bridge, when a call came through to our video Director, Lenny.

We all paused, and I took a sip of coffee…enjoying the beautiful view from where I was standing…the historical skyline…. drinking in how much I loved the project I was working on, the opportunity to be in such a beautiful place in the world, doing what I loved to do.

"Karen, the call is for you," Lenny said, carefully passing the phone to me. "It's your husband." I was immediately confused…Ralph never called me at work, unless it was urgent…let alone to an international location…. how did he get Lenny's phone number?

I tried to get all of these questions out before Ralph interrupted me. "Karen, I am so sorry to tell you this, but there's been a death in the family…"

My mind raced forward, as any Mother's would, first to my children. "Tell me the kids are ok." I said quickly. "They are fine." Ralph responded softly. With relief, I began a fast mental triage of my family. "Not my Dad…" I said, still not computing…he's so healthy… "

"No Karen…it's Cyndi. Cyndi died last night. They think it was a suicide."

I felt as if someone had hurled a softball into my chest. I couldn't breathe. It didn't compute. I couldn't understand.

Ralph said that there wasn't any more information yet, but that I was supposed to meet my Mom at the London Heathrow Marriott. They were booking us both a flight home that evening.

My kind London production crew helped me into a cab that would take me back to my hotel so I could quickly pack my things. My mind was numb as I took the ride, trying to piece together what could have happened to cause my sister to feel so lost and alone.

My heart broke thinking that I wasn't there for her to talk to...remembering our last in person conversation, just a little over a week before. I was at her house, with Lauren and Graham. They were swimming in Cyndi's pool with her sons, Devon and Ryan. It had been a beautiful day full of fun and laughter for the kids, but I remembered Cyndi's eyes. She was afraid. The divorce war was spiraling...and she was afraid of losing the fight...the house...the support for Ryan's teachers who were helping him with his Autism... but mostly of losing the kids completely. She knew her emotional health was unstable... but she was doing her best to hold everything together. But as usual, she diverted the conversation back to me, putting on her bright, chipper outlook, so I wouldn't focus on her situation. "Can't wait to hear everything about yours and Mom's trips when you get back...it's going to be amazing!"

As I was leaving, I reminded Cyndi that Ralph and I were there to help anyway way we could, and that we had more than enough room at our house if it ever came to her needing a place to stay. That day was July 3rd... I remember because it had been my Grandmother's birthday, and I had taken the ride back from Cyndi's to make a quick stop at her grave. As I got to the hotel to meet my mother, I said a quick prayer that Cyndi and my Grandmother were together.

It was a long, painful journey that followed. Painful, seeing the look on my Mother's face when hugged through sobs at the hotel. Painful calling my daughter Lauren, who was visiting her father in St. Louis, to tell her that her beloved

Aunt was gone. Painful seeing my father, and my siblings, and Cyndi's poor boys go through the wake and the funeral. Painful, as the oldest sibling, to be the one standing before the congregation, trying to explain to everyone there how much we loved her.

I remember sitting on the floor in my bedroom, just hours before the service, struggling to find the words to pay tribute to my beautiful sister. My heart was in a million pieces, I couldn't put two sentences together. I told Ralph that I didn't think I had the strength to do it. Suddenly, outside my window...I saw a butterfly go by...a symbol I remembered, was often associated with death and rebirth, and knew that meant that Cyndi was nearby. At that moment, my daughter Lauren came to show me the new dress she had picked out for the funeral...it was full of butterflies. Then my mother called, to let me know that she was able to get a small delivery of live butterflies, that we could release from the graveside.

With recharged energy knowing my sister was near, I was able to finish my speech. From the church podium, I could feel Cyndi's presence behind me. "Anyone who ever found themselves at the receiving end of Cyndi's kindness can tell you that her essence was shown in the little things she did...a warm dry towel waiting for you as you got out of the pool, a hug that held on just a bit longer when you were scared or lonely, the first cup of hot coffee out of the pot when you were exhausted, or a miniature Christmas tree that she made by hand. These are the things that love is really made of. For Cyndi, love was in the details. Yet, gratitude for any of these gifts almost embarrassed her. Kindness in her view was never something to be earned....it was the benefit you got just for knowing her. Coming from a big family whose members were always competing for center stage, Cyndi was content to dance around the perimeters of the spot-light and lead the applause for everyone else. She was the first to celebrate your success and be the bandleader for your joy...."

It felt so good to get those words out...even on one of the toughest days of our lives. I wanted more than anything for Cyndi to hear them, knowing that she would always be in our hearts.

A year, to the day, after Cyndi's passing, my Mom shared what she received in her journal from my sister. It was again, so representative of the love she was...always giving others and demonstrated in how she cared for all of us.

> *"As you go through this day, please remember the good times, the laughter and the love."* Cyndi wrote *"Just because the end of my life was so dark and tragic, don't color my life with tragedy.... I had my wonderful siblings, and my beautiful boys, and my dear loving parents. If I could have focused on that, my life would have taken a different course... remember the love we shared, not the pain and sorrow. It's only love that matters. Only love that crosses the divide of life and death, and only love that lives through eternity."*

My mother beautifully ends her book, tearfully acknowl-edging a beautiful butterfly that lands in front of her while visiting my sister's grave. Her final sentences sum the story of our family soul tribe's circle of grief. "None of this is about death," my Mother surmised. "All of this is about how love transcends all. Ours is a love story that deserved to be written, and I was the lucky one who became a pencil in God's hand."

Way to go, Momma.

LIFEMAPPING EXPLORATION #6 – Part 2

Lesson From
Your Squad
(Fear)

I'm so proud to share the story of my sister and our family's journey with you because I hope, as we get into the next part of this exercise, you too can see that "fear" situations, while often heartbreaking and painful, can offer you tremendous opportunities to grow.

There is an ancient Sufi prayer that says, "When the heart grieves for what is lost, the spirit rejoices over what is left." So, this can be as we face even our darkest fears.

My mother had every right to be bitter and angry, and could have chosen to blame God and the world for what happened to her daughter. Instead, she chose to face her grief, to dig deep within herself, to reach out to Cyndi and my Grandmother, transcending the belief that they were "gone" and out of reach of communication. And in doing so, she helped heal herself and created a memoir that has helped thousands of others with their grief in the process.

So, can it be for you, as you take this opportunity to examine those situations and relationships in your own life. Those who have brought you the most heartache have also brought you this same supreme opportunity to transcend your pain. To find some morsal of truth, lesson, hope and understanding so you can create a miracle of newfound understanding of the role they played in your world. You can be a mighty "sorcerer" in your own life. Like all the great wizards and magicians of old, you can summon the power of "source" (which is really just "love,") and completely reverse its meaning in your life.

As the great writer and spiritual activist Marianne Williamson once wrote, "we all have the power to be miracle workers..." I remember a quote from her unforgettable book, Return to Love, that always stayed with me. "A miracle is just a switch in perception from fear to love." And so, it is. We always have that opportunity to choose. It's what we applied to my journey from cancer to wellness with Graham, as well as my voyage from grief to belief with Cyndi. Those miracles have helped heal us all.

As so let us begin yours.

The Preface: The 4-7-8 Breathing Technique

As you begin this part of the exercise, I'd like you first to do a few minutes of breath work. Just to do a little bit of centering, and releasing, and heart chakra opening.

It will only take a few minutes. And this is an easy technique that you can do at any time. I just discovered this recently and I absolutely love the way it makes me feel. I really do forget to breathe, and this really helps me feel calm and energized at the same time.

What It Is

The 4-7-8 breathing technique requires a person to focus on taking a long, deep breath in and out.

Dr. Andrew Weil, a best-selling author and wellness physician, introduced this relaxation breathing exercise called the 4-7-8 breathing technique, which he believes can help with reducing anxiety, getting better sleep, among other great health benefits.

Here's how to do it:

Adopt a comfortable sitting position and place the tip of the tongue on the tissue right behind the top front teeth.

Now, focus on the following breathing pattern:

1. **For 4 seconds**: Breathe in quietly through the nose for count of 4 seconds
2. **For 7 seconds**: Hold your breath for count of 7 seconds
3. **For 8 seconds**: Exhale forcefully through the mouth, pursing the lips and making a "whoosh" sound, for a count of 8 seconds

Repeat the cycle up to 4 times.

I found doing that doing this exercise puts me in a wonderful centered place that allows all good ideas and feelings to come to me. Try it, I promise you will feel it!

Lifemapping Reminder: Before we start, a reminder of our grounding rules.

1. Give yourself a time limit – 15 minutes is a good goal for this exploration.
2. As in our prior exercises, find a comfortable location for you to do this work.
3. Try not to overthink it.
4. Be gentle with yourself – if this becomes too emotional for one sitting, you can divide this exercise into parts, or come back when you are ready.

Part Two: The "I AM" Lessons: Our Fear-Mates

As we did before, we are going to center this second part of the exercise on FEAR.... but rather than looking at the experiences themselves, we are focusing on the people who were some of the life-shapers on our journey.

Here is the process to follow: (details are on the next page)

- **Step 1: Identify** soul mates in Chapter 4 who were part of the more **fearful moments** in your life. Add their name to a circle.

- **Step 2: Evaluate** – How did this person make you feel?

- **Step 3: Actualize** Write the "I am" statement that translates what that person taught you about your own worthiness.

- **Step 4: Reflect** - Capture in your journal how these "I am statement" feel for you.

As before, I am including a sample here of my exercise from some of the key lessons from my Squad offered to me about fear.

MY SAMPLE EXERCISE:

	THINGS I HAVE LEARNED FROM MY FEAR SOUL SQUAD	
3rd Grade Teacher — Not Smart		High School Boy Friend — Too Nice
High School Counselor — Not Worthy	1. I am not smart enough 2. I am not talented enough 3. I am not pretty enough 4. I am not worth loving 5. I am insignificant	Post Divorce Boy Friend — Not honest
Ex-Husband — Betrayal	6. I am not creative 7. I am not articulate 8. I am not successful 9. I am not worthy of my dream	Friend — Not Loyal
Boss — No Leadership	10. I am not a good person 11. I am not committed enough 12. I am not strong enough 13. I am not worthy of loyalty 14. I am a not a good leader	Post Divorce Boy Friend — Not authentic
Work Associate — Selfishness	15. I am a failure 16. I am not brave enough 17. I am too nice 18. I am not paying attention to what's important 19. I am selfish	Another Boss — Judgement
College Professor — Failure	20. I am not dependable	Co-Worker — Jealousy

While it may be a difficult challenge to go through this list, I promise you, this will help you as you carve out your true purpose.

As you do this exercise, the purpose is for you to see what this person, who in some way signed up to be your "soul mate," was here to teach you. And chances are it is the very opposite of what you write down in your "I AM" statement.

Remember, both your love and fear squad are here to offer you opportunities to work through the things you came to learn. Your inner voice knows that these are not your truth, so we will identify them to shine a light on them so we can let them go. I can't wait to test this theory with you afterwards.

As you begin, I will leave you with another quote from the amazingly wise Marianne Williamson... *"Love is what we are born with. Fear is what we learn here."*

The form is for you on the next page, or you can use whatever format feels best for you.

EXERCISE: The "I AM" LESSONS FROM YOUR SQUAD: FEAR

- **Step 1: Identify** Go back to the list of the soul mates who you listed in your Lifemapping exercise in Chapter 4 who were part of the more **fearful moments** in your life. In each circle on the outside of your list, add their name.

- **Step 2: Evaluate** – Picture that person in your mind again. Relive some of those memories with them. How did this person make you feel?

- **Step 3: Actualize** – Write the "I am" statement that translates what that person taught you about your own worthiness. You can write more than one I am statement if there were multiple lessons that you learned from this person.

- **Step 4: Reflect** - When you have completed your list, take a few extra minutes to capture in your journal how these "I am" statements feel for you.

  - Do they surprise you?
  - Do they help you remember anything about yourself that you might have forgotten?
  - Do you believe them?

THINGS I HAVE LEARNED FROM MY FEAR SOUL SQUAD
1.
2.
3.
4.
5.
6.
7.
8.
9.
10.
11.
12.
13.
14.
15.
16.
17.
18.
19.
20.

Bringing Yourself Back to Center

Yuck. Feels disempowering, doesn't it? And a bit disconnected, too, isn't it? Because, as I look at my list...even now, I don't believe all those things about myself. And chances are, if I showed this list to anyone I work with or love, they would adamantly argue the opposite was true.

Does your list feel similar? Why are we so willing to believe and accept these inner voices and the opinions of these so-called self-chosen soul squads who have conjured so much angst and heartbreak into our lives?

As I broke down where some of my key teachers on the fear side came into my life... they came at the times when I was living in my moments of greatest self-doubt, from college classes to career to cancer. I let those inner voices talk me into my lack of confidence and self-esteem...to feelings of being judged, disconnected, powerless and defeated. My fear squad were there with a clear purpose... to help me see that I had disconnected from my own place of inner love...they came and reflected back at me my own fear, and dared me to see past the darkness.

Sometimes I did, but many times I didn't.

Who were some of the Fear mongers you identified in your Soul Squad? What were some of the things they said to you that became those voices of doubt, the negative chatter of "not enough-ness" in your head... that voice of the EGO that tried to pull you away from your pure and true state of love and enough-ness? What were the times that your intuition screamed at you to pay attention... but you listened instead to that other voice...when you hid behind your mask trying to hide the real you? And what were the times you let your inner voice talk you into believing those

FEAR "I am's" versus the LOVE one's you know in your heart are the essence of you.

Like Abraham Hicks once so wisely stated, **"A Belief is just a thought you keep thinking."**

You always have the power to choose what to believe.

LIFE MILESTONES: STEP 3 – Love & Fear & Self

OK – so we are back to another "moment of truth…"

Now that you've done your Love and Fear Squad Assessment, we're again going to take a moment to place them side by side.

Again, I've shared mine below, to give you a sense of the irony of the story it tells.

THINGS I LEARNED FROM MY LOVE SQUAD	THINGS I LEARNED FROM MY FEAR SQUAD
1. I am a storyteller	1. I am not smart enough
2. I am unconditionally loved	2. I am not talented enough
3. I love unconditionally	3. I am not pretty enough
4. I am a talented writer/storyteller/producer	4. I am not worth loving
5. I am a mentor/supporter	5. I am insignificant
6. I am creative/creator	6. I am not creative
7. I am kind	7. I am not articulate
8. I am an uplifter	8. I am not successful
9. I am wise	9. I am not worthy of my dream
10. I am intuitive	10. I am not a good person
11. I am a teacher	11. I am not committed enough
12. I am a achiever	12. I am not strong enough
13. I am brave	13. I am not worthy of loyalty
14. I am persistent	14. I am not a good leader
15. I am loyal	15. I am a failure
16. I am an inspirational leader	16. I am not brave enough
17. I am a visionary	17. I am too nice
18. I am an innovator	18. I am not paying attention to what's important
19. I am a seeker	19. I am selfish
20. I am believer	20. I am not dependable

The most amazing thing you will find as you compare your lists is that for so many of your key insights, things that you thought they taught you, completely contradict each other. Take a look when I map them side by side.

LESSONS FROM MY SQUAD The Contradictions Corner	
LOVE	**FEAR**
LOVE #2 - I am unconditionally loved	FEAR #4 - I am not worth loving
LOVE #4 - I am talented	FEAR #2 - I am not talented
LOVE #6 - I am creative	FEAR #6 - I am not creative
LOVE #7 - I am persistent	FEAR #13 - I am not committed enough
LOVE #17 - I am a visionary	FEAR #9 - I am not worthy of my dream
LOVE #15 - I am an inspirer	FEAR #5 - I am full of self-doubt

Like the exercise in chapter 6, this again tells a story of self-contradictions. How can we know such two completely different versions of ourselves? It all depends on who we are willing to believe.

Take a moment and do the same thing with your two lists and tee up the Contradictions? The Similarities? Were there the same learnings from your Milestone Lists, as Well as your Soul Squad lists?

LIFE MILESTONES: Love or Fear The Contradictions Corner	
LOVE	**FEAR**

So now...the big reveal. You ready? We are going to line up all of the boxes, from our last Chapters work, as well as this one's and line them up.

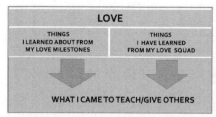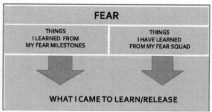

Take a moment to really look carefully at the story that is lining up for you under these boxes. Everything.... I mean everything on the side of LOVE is always TRUTH...everything on the side of FEAR are FALSEHOODS...trying to talk us out of our TRUTH.

And herein, lies the beginning of the meaning of your Soul's Purpose. What have you come to give from your truest authentic self...? Your I AM LOVE self? And what are the untruths you are being told, or are you telling yourself, that you just need to let go of? In the end, in its simplest form, Your Love Milestones show you what you have come to Give/Teach others, and your Fear Milestones show you what you have come to Learn/Release.

Did you get a sense of recognition of yourself with the exercise? Are any of these insights beginning to ring true for you? Does it help you begin to see yourself in a different way?

The focus of our work in the next Chapter will be to absorb and embrace these learnings from your past so you can begin to see how to apply them to what you love to do.... which is another hint to help you unravel your LifeMap.

Soul Release Exercise

Let's finish up this incredible work by taking a moment to release some of the residual awareness weight you may be still feeling around our solar plexus (that's the chakra, or energy center, where all the self-judgement and criticism resides).

Can you feel it? It's that place just under your heart at the middle lower part of your ribcage. It's what I always feel when "my inner self" needs protection. To bring myself back to alignment, I like to do a release exercise by giving thanks to those who have offered me this opportunity to learn.

Here's how to do it:

Deep breath in…. deep breath out. And again…. deep breath in…deep breath out (I promise I am doing this right along with you.)

In your mind, picture one of those Fear-mates who may have ended up playing a role on your "I am…" list. Instead of reliving the moment that may have wronged you… picture them in their own state of Fear. What things have they might have gone through in their own life experience that they may have been projecting on to you?

Was it a boss who may have intimidated you, to deflect his own inner insecurity? Is it possible that they **did you a favor** by firing you, or making you so uncomfortable that you had to look for another job?

Was it a lover who was unfaithful to you because of some deeper, unmet need within themselves? Recognize that they **did you a favor** by actually leaving you…to open you up to a better version of love.

Was it a friend or co-worker that might have betrayed you, or lied about you for their own gain? They **did you a favor** by re-instating your own sense of integrity and honesty, and reminding you to never do what they did to you to another person.

No matter how deep the wound, there is an opportunity to see hidden "favor" behind the mates who seemingly inflicted their pain upon us.

Here's a chance to thank them for **"doing you that favor...."**

I want you to say to yourself, out loud, or in your journal, however it feels best, about those one or two people.

> "I forgive and release (NAME) for (WHAT THEY DID) because I know that we were brought together to learn (LESSON). I know and see that they are part of my soul squad and recognize how they offered me an equal opportunity to choose love over fear.
>
> I thank (NAME) for the role that they played in the journey of my life, and lovingly forgive and release them lovingly from my past. I see them for the light that they are, and the soul mates we have become in this lifetime. I am grateful for their role, and now embrace them only from a place of love."

If you can do this exercise for just one or two people from your squad and visualize them thanking you for your mutual role on the life journey, you will help release the lock of that experience on your heart and open it back to love.

Well, that was quite the journey. We opened this chapter with a quote from Mother Teresa...that sums up beautifully the understanding that the souls we encounter in our lives can be blessing or lessons. I would say, that they can be both. When those lessons have seemed their hardest and you just need to get past the people who have participated in this learning with you, I offer you this great poem that has also been attributed to Mother Teresa. It has helped me often during some of my darkest moments. No matter what definition you give your "God," be it "Heavenly Father" or "Mother Gaia" or "Source," I offer this here as a resource to also help you let go, knowing that there is always a higher meaning...and that is YOU.

"People are often unreasonable, irrational, and self-centered.
Forgive them anyway.

If you are kind, people may accuse you of selfish, ulterior motives.
Be kind anyway.

If you are successful, you will win some unfaithful friends and some genuine enemies.
Succeed anyway.

If you are honest and sincere people may deceive you.
Be honest and sincere anyway.

What you spend years creating, others could destroy overnight.
Create anyway.

If you find serenity and happiness, some may be jealous.
Be happy anyway.

The good you do today, will often be forgotten.
Do good anyway.

Give the best you have, and it will never be enough.
Give your best anyway.

In the final analysis, it is between you and God.
It was never between you and them anyway.

—Mother Teresa"

SOUL GOODY BAG

Here are some resources mentioned in this chapter for you for further exploration:

- **Many Lives, Many Masters by Dr. Brian Weiss** - As a traditional psychotherapist, Dr. Brian Weiss was astonished and skeptical when one of his patients began recalling past-life traumas that seemed to hold the key to her recurring nightmares and anxiety attacks. With more than one million copies in print, *Many Lives, Many Masters* is one of the breakthrough texts in alternative psychotherapy and remains as provocative and timeless as it was when first published.

- **Only Love is Real: The Story of Two Soulmates Reunited By Dr. Brian Weiss** –Elizabeth and Pedro are unaware that they have been lovers throughout the long centuries -- until fate brings them together again. This is a story of the meaning of soul mates.

- **Celestial Conversations: Healing Relationships After Death by Lo Anne Mayer.** One morning Lo Anne Mayer wrote a letter to her mother, who had died a year earlier. Despondent over the strained relationship they had endured in life, Mayer started the journal because she still longed for healing. So began a remarkable soul-to-soul correspondence that restored their bond. When her own daughter died, Mayer started a new journal that soothed her grief. Now she shares her story and simple technique with bereaved people everywhere.

- **Return to Love by Marianne Williamson** – This mega-bestselling spiritual guide shares Marianne's reflections on *A Course in Miracles* along with her insights on how love is a potent force, the key to inner peace, and how by practicing love we can make our own lives more fulfilling while creating a more peaceful and loving world for our children.

- **Michelle Brock** - Michelle Brock is a New York City based spiritual development life coach who specializes in past life regression. She is also an intuitive counselor, a psychic medium, a master hypnotist, and has studied spirituality, shamanism, meditation, divination, astrology, and energy medicine techniques from many different world traditions. She can be reached on her website at **Michelle-brock.com**

SECTION TWO

WHERE YOU ARE: YOUR LIFEMAPPING JOURNEY TODAY

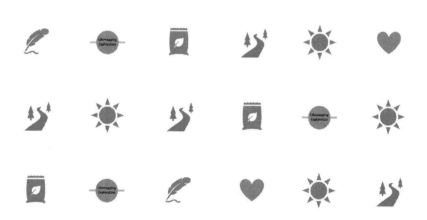

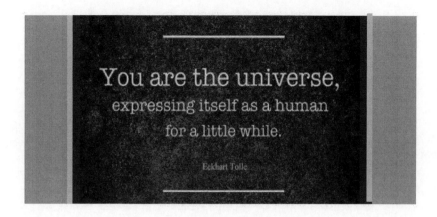

You are the universe,
expressing itself as a human
for a little while.

Eckhart Tolle

CHAPTER 8

EMBRACING YOUR PURPOSE

In November of 2014, I was working at my desk at AT&T, when a friend of mine peeked in the door of my office. With a mischievous grin on her face, she asked "Hey Karen, you're a runner, aren't' you?

Looking up from my work, seeing my teammate grinning with expectation, I sensed an ultimatum coming.

Shiz was headed up our Corporate Sponsorships team... she was a brilliant, outgoing and full of infectious positive energy that was catapulting her up the corporate ladder like a rocket. She and I had become fast friends when I started my new advertising role in Dallas, and she was the first person to take me out for a real Texas margarita when I arrived.

Shiz leaned carefully on the glass door of my office, arms crossed, grinning at me.

"Oh my gosh girl, what the heck are you up to?" I countered, knowing this was not going to end well for me. Shiz only asked questions when she already knew the answers.

"I'm here to offer you the opportunity of a lifetime," she said, with her Texas twang twirling with sass.

"There it is," I responded. "Why do I feel like this is more like you're 'making me an offer that I can't refuse.'"

"It IS…"Shiz affirmed, jumping to the office chair next to me. "So here it is. How would you like to run the Boston Marathon in April? I've got two spots left."

It turned out that since AT&T was a prime sponsor of the event, it was able to offer the opportunity to a few employees to run in the 4th wave of the race. "So, you don't have to officially qualify, Karen," Shiz said.

"Well dang," I thought, eliminating that possibility. That said, the run was still 26.2 miles. My daily average was about three?

I quickly dismissed the idea. There was no way. I had just managed to survive my turning 50 crisis and was quite happy lying low, embracing my ever-comfortable status quo.

"Shiz, darling…" I laughed. "I'm a jogger, not a runner. I've never done a marathon." I finished the sentence in my head with "…and I never will."

"C'mon girl. Even I'm gonna do it. And look at me…" her hands swept around her stomach, landing on her hips. "I'm going to have to train big!! C'mon, just think about it, I mean who gets to run the Boston Marathon? This is an opportunity of a lifetime!" That triggered one of those little knowing voices in my head, but I said nothing, now very frightened over the prospect of what I now knew was inevitable.

"My work is done here," Shiz said, satisfied with her hand-iwork. "I can see those wheels turning. I'll be back tomorrow to ask you again."

And that, my friends is how the universe works...when it wants you, it comes knocking at your door.

Five months later, I was on a school bus, jammed packed with runners from all over the world heading for the town of Hopkinton Mass, where the 26.2-mile Boston Marathon begins. As we sped down the highway, for what seemed like hours away from downtown Boston, I was certain I had made the biggest mistake of my life.

That year was the first race after the Boston Marathon bombing, so there was a definite edge in the air that lay-ered over the surge of adrenalin that everyone was already feeling. Patriotic intensity and anticipation filled us, even as we took note of the squads of police and S.W.A.T. teams on top of the surrounding buildings, as we made our way to the starting line.

Shiz gave me a wink as we started off, but I quickly lost her in the sea of runners, at first barely able to shuffle ahead in the vast denseness of the pack. But our muddled mass, quickly thinned into a pulsing river of bibbed num-bers, covering the streets and bobbing around corners, and something took over within me. I slowly felt my body relax and become one, heartbeat to heartbeat, with other souls who were on their own quests, their own once in a lifetime, marathon moments.

Almost immediately, I was mesmerized by the crowd of bystanders stacked three to four people deep, with their signs and cowbells, cheering us on. Some of us had written our names with a black sharpie marker on our arms, and so when we passed, they would call to us with their rallying shouts as we passed. "Way to go Karen!!!" "You can do this

Karen!!" "So proud of you Karen." You're Boston Strong Karen!! "Their voices were like a steady drum beat of energy and connection. As the miles fell away, I felt at one with every runner, every person on every street corner. I held back tears of both pride in myself and of gratitude for this rally of pure human spirit.

When I finally turned the corner onto Boylston Street, I got a glimpse of the beautiful yellow and blue lettering of the finish line. Unlike the rest of my competitors who were picking up their pace to push their final run times, I slowed down to drink in the magic of what I knew was nearing the end of my once-in-a-lifetime experience. The crowd was still full of energy, even at the end of the race where the winning marathon runners had already crossed hours before. They were still there in the thousands waiting for us, as I high fived the bellowing crowd savoring what it felt like to be embraced by the magic of that moment. I didn't want it to end! Later, I hugged Shiz who found me in the crowd, full of smiles and sweat. "Did I call it?" she asked, reading the answer on my flushed face, smiling so hard it hurt.

This marked my new beginning. It began a marathon to the next leg of my journey, which would inspire me to take on my biggest challenge yet.

The Next Step in Your Journey Begins Here

Now that you've completed the inventory of your love and fear milestones, and recognize the key influencers on your soul squad, you're ready to map the next layer that will truly help reveal your purpose. Where you are today.

Your soul squad and milestones are part of the foundation of your story. They are evidence of the accomplishments of the plan you put in place before you started this lifetime.

But there is more to your soul contract than the people and experiences you chose to help you learn.

The next two Chapters of your Soul Mapping Journey are all about embracing the NOW.... the PRESENT moment on your lifemap and embracing what you love.

Think of this section as the icing on your spiritual soul cake.

Welcome to Chapter 8

Embracing Your Purpose will take all of the amazing work we've done in the last few chapters and help you identify your mission. What you came **"to be."**

This Lifemapping layer will help you begin to fill in the color of the map of you, by highlighting **your talents and interests**, your inner GPS that points to your soul's north star. Now with the understanding you have gained from your milestones and soul squad, this section will provide that third dimension of yourself, to help you see how your past led you to your present, which will be the map of your future.

Here you will receive the tools to help you stand in your truth, by asking **3 Magical Questions** that will let your heart speak. This will identify the real spark of your purpose... which is about how to actualize what you've come to learn and give, **it's about what you are here to do."**

This is the space where you can step away from your personal history **and take a plunge into the delicious present.** We'll dive into the "beingness" of where your feet are right now, yes, right now...no I mean right now!!...so you can harness the power you have power over, which is the power of the *present moment*.

This is how we'll invite your precious inspiration back into your life...and provide precious, soul-filling time to listen within, banishing the darkening doubt so you can reawaken into the today-light.

Here's the plan:

1. We'll learn about the "power of now" and how to harness it as a jumping off point to find and understand our purpose.
2. We'll explore the differences between our inner and outer purpose, and how ego gets in the way of us truly finding what makes us happy.
3. We'll jump into the 3 Magic Questions that will help you identify your own unique talents and gifts, just by thinking about the things you enjoy doing.
4. We 'll create your customized Designer Dream statement, that reflects everything you are and have been born to be!

Let's do this!

The Ego and the Power of Now

There is arguably no more famous teacher on how to awaken your life's purpose than the contemporary spiritual writer and teacher Eckhart Tolle. At the age of 29, an intense inner transformation, which some would call a "spiritual awakening," radically changed the course of his life. Those learnings would become the foundation of his best-selling books, "The Power of Now", and "A New Earth", which would inspire millions with his profound yet simple teachings on how to use the power of the present moment to connect and understand our highest selves.

"It is not uncommon for people to spend their whole life waiting to start living." Eckhardt writes in the Power of Now. "As soon as you honor the present moment, all unhappiness and struggle dissolve, and life begins to flow with joy and ease. When you act out the present-moment awareness, whatever you do becomes imbued with a sense of quality, care, and love."

This idea of living in the now was a wakeup call for me. When I started taking mental inventory of my thoughts, I was astounded by how many of them revolved around something that had happened in the past (something I regretted, something I forgot to do, a memory of an experience I wish I could change) or something coming up (an errand I needed to do, an email I needed to write, a meeting I was going to have). When did I ever really just sit in the present moment and fully appreciate the full power that it offered me to control WHAT I thought about and the EMOTION that I felt with that thought? It all went back to the power of the emotional scale, and yet, I'd say 99% of the time, I overlooked that control I had over my present moment, and thereby, the direction those thoughts were taking me.

Eckart also introduced me to the idea that I was not alone in my head...and that I shared my inner space with a powerful "ego." I always thought of ego as a bad word that was associated with being self-centered and self-absorbed, or having a superior attitude. It was a word you'd use to label someone who was full of themselves...who put themselves above others.

But Tolle's definition of the ego is different. He describes it as that inner voice that judges, complains, and has opinions. Ego is the measure of you against everyone else. It is our inner monkey mind that defines and separates us from others, and it keeps us from connecting to our real selves, our source...which is love.

In other words, the ego is the great impostor. Ego is fear.

This present, is the present moment, where Eckhart says is our place of power, because it is where our past ends and our future begins. "**Most humans are never fully present** in the **now**," he says, "Because unconsciously they believe that the next moment must be **more** important than this one. But then you miss your whole life, which is **never** not **now**."

The decision to make the present into your friend, is the end of the ego." Tolle writes "Realize deeply that the present moment is all you ever have. **Make the Now the primary focus of your life**."

This concept offers us our next big shift on our Lifemapping journey. We have bravely done our personal inventory of looking lovingly back at our past and all the soul-purposeful reasons that we have reached our current destination. But our next steps are turn for the moment away from that knowledge and to drink in the now. To fully embrace the moment of where we are to feel what calls us. That according to Eckhart is "where our true power lies."

Understanding the Difference Between Inner Purpose and Outer Purpose

Eckhardt's words are deep, spiritual, and at times so rich, that they take multiple times re-reading to understand. But at their core, his message explains how we can free ourselves from the past, live more fully in the present, and come to the calm, joyful place where intuition, creativity, and wisdom lives.

Eckhardt says that the key to a really fulfilled life is when our **outer purpose** aligns with our **inner purpose**. The outer purpose is the things we do, our careers, our vocations, the things we do day by day. Our inner purpose is the opposite...it not a state of action...it's not about setting a future goal...it's about being content, accepting, and at ease with where we are and who we are, right now...with no assigned outcome or expectation. We are not in a state of wanting and looking at the things that have not yet manifested ...but instead, we are connected to our inner light and harmony,

We are at one with our human being-ness versus our human doing-ness.

To Be, or Not To Be...That is the Question

There is no better example of someone "living in the moment" than my friend Allison Feehan. She is another one of those courageous seekers, who was able to head the sound of her own inner voice, and cast off all of the "shoulds" of the outer world's expectations and follow the star of her own heart.

And as for all seekers, who answer the call to find their soul's purpose, Allison too faced many mountains along the way. She actually came very close to taking Shakespeare's quote to a grim reality, where her "being" almost was "not to be" when the birth of her child threw life out of balance. But in doing so, "a new earth" of her own emerged, and life forever changed for her and her family.

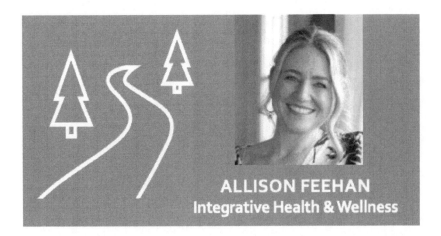

ALLISON FEEHAN
Integrative Health & Wellness

My life changed the day I entered the hospital for the birth of my child, but not in the way that I expected. I was admitted without delay and hooked up to the necessary equipment to monitor my vitals and those of the baby, who had been in the breech position for 32 weeks in utero. The plan was to manually turn the baby or schedule a cesarean if the baby did not move into the birthing position before it was time.

Hours later, my labor is not progressing as well as the doctor had hoped. My child was in the proper position, but no ultrasound caught the fact that the umbilical cord was wrapped several times around the baby's throat.

Not only was my child in distress but I too ran into trouble. My blood pressure rose at an accelerated rate with no sign of coming down. With the two of us in a life-or-death situation, my husband was facing the terrible decision of who to save. Through my oxygen mask and tears I begged my husband to choose the baby.

In a last effort and some quick decisions, the doctor agreed to let me try one push but, if it didn't work, they would have to do an emergency c-section. With every ounce of what I imagined might be my last breath, I visualized myself pushing what felt like a refrigerator up a flight of stairs ... I'll never forget the doctor's words as I gasped for air, "I don't believe it" he said.

My child's head was crowned and, within minutes, he was free! It would take hours for both of us to be completely out of the woods, but that was the life-changing moment that taught me the real test of love and fear.

There was no doubt that my love for my child surpassed the fear of losing my own life. It was an easy decision. In that instant, I realized it would have been ok for me to let go. I thought perhaps my time here had been fulfilled and the Universe and spirit needed me more on the "other side." Trusting in the plan of what should be and not having control over a frightful situation led me to truly TRUST the Universe and the bigger plan already decided for us. The plan we put in place prior to this lifetime.

This realization is now how I live my life every day. My life's purpose is to be here – to be a Mother, a Light to those that need it, and a healer of mind, body, and spirit. I wouldn't be able to do this if this experience didn't open my eyes to the importance of my purpose.

That is when I also realized that I needed to stop pretending my gift didn't exist. I've been a psychic and medium since I was four years old and avoided using that gift out of fear. I kept everything that I intuitively saw and knew to myself, even from my husband. It can feel *uncomfortable to be different sometimes. But after my near-death experience with my son's birth, it occurred to me that being different was why I was here.*

As my children grew up, I started to share more and more of my intuitive messages with my husband. Once my children went into middle school, I decided to start my own practice and began my work in holistic health, energy healing and intuitive work, including spiritual coaching.

I decided to leave my corporate job and be in-service to others. I decided I wanted to make life changing impacts on my clients and the world. I knew that I needed to help others get in touch with their purpose, to help them move through their pain and traumas, to help them understand why they are here, and the very special magic that they too hold.

My life has forever changed since I made that decision and the countless messages and feedback, I received on how I changed people's lives has been worth it all. Connecting to the very source that put us here on this planet is available to all of us. We just have to connect to it and not be afraid to do so.

Allison is a true seekers story about finding true meaning by facing our deepest fears. Her courage to live in her truth and share the gifts that she has been given is now helping hundreds to heal, find hope and live healthier lives. She is an example of how living in the moment of being and sharing of all she is, has helped her find and embrace her life's purpose.

To be…. without question.

Doing the Now: AKA Don't Forget to Take Time to Smell the Roses

Sound impossible to be so "Zen?"

Try an experiment with me. These are little ways you can condition yourself to find the "now" in your everyday experiences.

Let's do the now thing now...ready?

1. **What Do I Observe?** Stop what you are doing right now and take a long careful look at your hands. Observe the back of them: your knuckles, your fingernails, the veins leading from your arms carrying blood below your skin. Flip your hands over and look at your palms, the lifelines, the different color and texture of your skin, your fingertips that carry the unique imprint of you. Without straining, relaxed but alert, give your complete attention to your hands...every detail of them. Can you observe without the voice in your head taking over? Can you keep your attention there for a full minute without your thoughts drifting away to other things?

2. **What Do I Feel?** Let's continue focusing on your hands, now bringing in the sensation of feeling. Rub your hands together, intertwining your fingers.... slowly massaging each finger, the muscles under your thumbs, the bones around your wrists. Feel the how the tension is soothed as you rub the stress out of the tendons, around your delicate joints and fingertips...appreciating this small conscious act of self-care for yourself, and the feeling of the **aliveness of the body** you are in.

3. **What Do I Experience?** Take a moment and look at your hands as part of your body. Observe your surroundings...the hands connected to the body that is present in a place. Feel the seat beneath you, your feet on the floor, the temperature of the room. Your **presence in the space** that you are in. Try not to analyze the space but take account of the physicality of your environment. Is there furniture in the room, a window? Are you on a plane or train? Just BE where you are. Give your complete attention to everything you see without thoughts or judgement. Take account of the fact that YOU ARE where you are, right now.

The idea of this exercise is to try to catch yourself as often as possible and STOP, to condition yourself to slow down and appreciate the present. Doing these little actions that "catch yourself" and bring you back to the now is the first step in helping you to live a more consciously.

"Give your complete attention to what you feel, and refrain from mentally labeling it." Says Tolle in "The Power of Now," "Stay alert, stay present — with your whole Being, with every cell of your body. As you do so, you are bringing a light into this darkness. This is the flame of your consciousness."

Ah...starting to feel the Zen now.... you?

This is something that I have tried to practice more and more, because it helps me "tune in" to how I'm feeling. Often, when I can get outside in the sunlight...I try to really focus on the feeling of that warmth on my face, the beauty of the sky, the smell of the air, the safety of my feet on the ground. That tapping into the moment connects me with my gratitude.

"You are never more essentially, more deeply, yourself than when you are still," Tolle writes in A New Earth. "When you are still, you are who you were before you temporarily assumed this physical and mental form is called a person. You are who you will be when the form dissolves. When you are still, you are who you are beyond your temporal existence: Consciousness-unconditioned, formless, eternal." (P.256 ANE)

Now that you have a sense of what this "being in the moment" feels like, I'd like to introduce you to my dear Life-mapper friend, Marie. Like most of us, Marie had lived in a way that she thought was "on purpose," making choices that she thought were right for herself and her family. But as you'll see when she describes how when she got to this point in the Lifemapping exercise, it became clear that her inner purpose was missing...and this was the place where her journey to self- understanding really began.

LIFEMAPPER STORIES

MARIE'S STORY: Finding the Future in the Present

Marie was quiet through the beginning of the Lifemapping Workshop. She had signed up at the request of a friend, and I could tell from her energy that dedicating a three-hour afternoon to digging into her soul-story was not exactly her idea of a good time. That said, she listened patiently as I explained the plan for the class, and went right to work on the first exercise, mapping out her key milestones.

As the group began to share their feedback, Marie hung back. When I asked her if she wanted to share any of her own insights, she shyly smiled. "You know, my life is just normal," she said. "I come from a great family. I now have a great family of my own...but there really aren't a lot of big 'aha' moments on my list. I just don't think I'm one of those people who is supposed to have this big life full of a lot of extreme experiences and lessons. And I'm ok with that. It's really good enough."

I smiled back at Marie...seeing her so clearly as an earlier version of myself. Her words said one thing, but her energy conveyed another.

"I totally get that Marie..." I said (because I really did). "But when you say the words, 'it's good enough' out-loud. What does that feel like?

Marie shrugged, and then smiled, understanding where I was headed.

"There is nothing wrong with something being "good," I said. "When I ask a friend how they are doing, and they say, "I'm good," it communicates a certain level of contented emotion to it. But when you add the word "enough," it subtly feels like your good bar slides down a bit, don't you think? It's like you've just barely managed to make the mark. Good enough, is not the same as good. "

"Let's do this," I suggested. "Let's go through your time-line now, so we can see how you got here.... I want to get you to a place where you can look at these from the perspective of your inner purpose, which I think might surprise you."

Skeptically, Marie nodded. "Game on!!" I thought.... my FAVORITE part of this was being able to show people WAYYYY more about themselves than they can see through their own life lens.

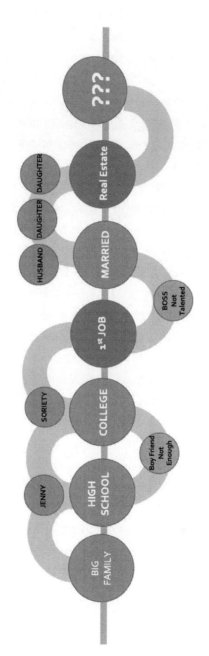

MARIE's Life Map

LOVE/CONNECTION

FEAR/DISCONNECTION

BIG FAMILY

JENNY

HIGH SCHOOL

Boy Friend Not Enough

SORIETY

COLLEGE

1st JOB

BOSS Not Talented

HUSBAND

DAUGHTER

DAUGHTER

MARRIED

Real Estate

???

What we uncovered in Marie's milestones, not surprisingly, was she was more than enough. Marie's life was, indeed, all about the doing, and the level of her authentic self that she brought to everything she did.

When we looked back upon her childhood, her family, high school and college experiences, Marie was animated and happy. As often the case, more milestones came to the surface as she recalled her early activities, filling in her thin outline, with deep friendships, her cheerleading squad, her family trips to the Jersey shore. It was also pretty clear that Marie had a strong sense of self, that was anchored in a loving desire to be of service to others.

"Being the fourth child in a family of six, teaches you pretty quickly to define yourself," Marie laughed, "Otherwise, you just blend in with the crowd."

She laughed as she shared a story about when she was six, and how she was left behind after a family trip to the shore. "My parents had driven about 15 minutes before they realized that I was missing," Marie recalled. "And it sounds funny now, but I never quite got over that...I always had this subtle fear that if I didn't make my voice counted, somehow I would be left behind."

When she got out of college, Marie went on to become a paralegal assistant, supporting a female legal executive at a New York City publishing firm. But instead of being mentored by her powerful boss, Marie was treated as a subservient caretaker, required to work long nights and weekends. "It was so disappointing," Marie recalled about her former boss. "She was a brilliant, hardworking lawyer, recognized by her male piers as a powerful force in the court room...but behind closed doors, she was an insecure alcoholic who used me to cover up her tracks."

While the judgement sounded harsh, I could tell it came from a place of great personal pain for Marie's past. She went on to take several other roles in the business world, but they were equally unfulfilling. Marie quickly realized that working within the confines of a defined corporate structure left her feeling empty and uninspired.

Her role as a wife and a mother of two daughters, however, brought in a newfound sense of purpose and joy. "I realized as a mom, that I was being loved and needed for who I was...my role evolved out of that, from the inside out really, instead of the outside in."

Still, the accomplishments of everyone around her seemed monumental compared to her own. Her siblings were all rising up the corporate ladder, following shiny careers with big salaries. She lived in a neighborhood that placed a high value on success, and home values, and material wealth. It was hard to stay balanced in the social game of "have's and have nots."

Still, she kept lightening focused on her family. As Marie's girls grew up, she became active in the school system, organizing activities and events, that ultimately led to her becoming head of the PTA and then the school board. She got to know the other parents, educators and administrators in town. She branched out her career roots and became a real estate agent, that helped further intwine deeper relationships with families that were both coming and going into town. Marie was in fact, living in her now, not working for the "resume" but from a place of broader service for her neighbors and for her community.

That's where Marie got her first aha moment. She began to see that all the fulfillment she was receiving from her life stemmed from her authentic connection with her inward sense of purpose...it came from her family...and the love and light within.

All she needed was to re-examine her life through a different lens...from the NOW. She was able to shift her view and see she really was living a life that was right on purpose. She was just evaluating her accomplishments from other's perspectives of success versus her own.

"The great arises out of small things that are honored and cared for," Tolle writes. "The present moment is always small in the sense that it is always simple but concealed within it lies the greatest power." (ANE p.266)

Creating Our Lives on Purpose

Like Marie, we all, in some way, spend our lives trying to define our inner purpose by taking action. Like me signing up for that marathon, finding that spark of meaning can start with a shift in our focus...of redefining what we think we can or can't do. It can start by saying yes to the unexpected opportunities, insights and inspirations that come our way.

This is what I like to call, listening to the "heartstrings of your soul" – the notes and sounds that make up your own unique symphony.... the opus of your life's work. Right now, you may feel like you are coming from the place of the unknown to the "now known," the YOU that you didn't quite see or understand before.

But now, with the knowledge of the power you have to be fully present in your life, and seeing where your feet may have stepped in the direction of love or fear, let's deliberately create your new now to create the future (quite literally) of your dreams.

How does that sound? Ah...like an Opus my dear one... like an Opus!!!

Finding Your Life's Opus

In the 1995 film, "Mr. Holland's Opus," Richard Dreyfuss plays the role of Glenn Holland, an aspiring composer who takes a job as a high school music teacher to pay the rent and support his growing family. As he continues to work on his lifelong dream of writing his great symphony, the years pass. After 30 years of teaching music, Mr. Holland is let go from his job, and his students come back to pay a surprise orchestrated tribute to the impact he has had on all of their lives.

One of those students, Gertrude Lang, had lost her way before joining Mr. Holland's music class, returns to lead the celebration. She is now the state Governor. Her words tell the story of Mr. Holland had unknowingly lived his inner purpose, and it has had very little to do with writing his symphony.

"Mr. Holland has had a profound influence on my life and on a lot of lives I know. But I have a feeling that he considers a great part of his own life misspent. Rumor had it he was always working on this symphony of his. And this was going to make him famous, rich, probably both. But Mr. Holland isn't rich, and he isn't famous, at least not outside of our little town. So, it might be easy for him to think himself a failure. But he would be wrong, because I think that he's achieved a success far beyond riches and fame. Look around you. There is not a life in this room that you have not touched, and each of us is a better person because of you. We are your symphony, Mr. Holland. We are the melodies and the notes of your opus. We are the music of your life."

How many of us do not have any idea of the lives we have touched or impacted? How many of us get to a point in our lives where we feel that our lives may have been misspent, or that we have not achieved a level of "greatness" that we'd had planned on? This story that almost ends on a broken dream, but instead, uncovers and shines a light on an inspired life with an unseen ripple effect impacting the lives of many. It's a story that reminds us that we never can fully know the effect our lives can fully have on another... and as we all work so carefully to craft and construct our daily lives around the visions of goals and achievements that we think are our dreams, we may not realize that they are, in fact, already unfolding all around us.

"What the world will not tell you...is that you cannot **become success**," writes Tolle, "you can only **be successful.**" And that my friend comes from living successfully from the present moment.

My goal for this Lifemapping experience, is for you to see the impact you have already made on this world with what you have already done, and now apply those learnings to see the YOU of TODAY, to get you to the place where you can EXPAND that LOVE to be ALL THAT YOU ALREADY ARE.

Once you see this, your OPUS will unfold.

As we embark on this last self-inventory exercise, you'll identify where your "power of now" lies... at that is within the heartstrings of your soul. These are the things that call to you...that are the color in between the lines of your life. The details that make you unique, special, individual, one of a kind...classic.

They are your talents, your passions, your joys, your most actualized vision of yourself.

And, so too...as every symphony – there are flats and sharps, minors and majors, harmonies and solos... it is what makes each composition truly beautiful and unique. It's what moves us to dance, to sing, to cry.

As Eckart Tolle said, "**Be true to life by being true to your inner purpose. As you become present, and thereby total in what you do, your actions will be charged with spiritual power.**" It is one of the keys to manifesting everything we desire.

This is how we will approach this next exercise.

This goes against everything we've ever learned, doesn't it? Haven't we all been told that our life should be laser focused and goal-oriented, geared to a resume of carefully calculated plans. Isn't it all about getting the A's? Actions, Accomplishments, Acquisitions, Achievements, Accolades?

Ah, but the universe will show you that the opposite is true.

For so many of us, we are already living our life's purpose and we just don't know it. For so many of the people who have looked at their life maps, it took this vital step for them to break through what they thought were their life's expectations and instead reframe their life experiences to see the true vision of their purpose.

As Marie showed us earlier, she was one of them. But now she was in a place where she wanted to learn more. "I want to take this inner sense of purpose that I do have and do more with it," she said. "I want to take a leap into something more." In other words, step out of the comfort zone into the truth zone.

This is the exercise that really helped Marie turn the corner. Welcome to the marathon Marie

As always, let us begin our inner journey with a centering thought:

SOULFIRMATION #8

"Today, I embrace my intention to be in the present moment
I live my life from the point of view of my inner purpose
That shines through
Creating the manifestations of my outer purpose
The true evidence of my creative intentions.
It is here I will come to the know
Who I am
And all I intended to be...
I am a spark of limitless source
connected always to my power within."

LIFEMAPPING EXPLORATION #7

Embracing Your Purpose

Listening to the Language of your heart

Before I wrote a single word of this book, my amazing publisher Melanie Warner, gave me an exercise. She challenged me to answer three questions. She promised that if I answered them honestly, that they would show me what I was supposed to write about.

Doing this exercise really opened my eyes and inspired me to add this third layer to my Lifemapping exploration work. It's helped so many people in my workshops connect the dots on not only understanding how their milestones and squad have shaped them, but that the answers to their life's purpose were already in the desires and dreams living within their heart...they just needed a voice.

Sound too good to be true? Well, let's test it and see for yourself.

Lifemapping Reminder:

1. Give yourself a time limit – 15 minutes is a good goal for this exploration.
2. As in our prior exercises, find a comfortable location for you to do this work.
3. Try not to overthink it.

In this exercise, your only assignment is to have fun! This is the place where you recognize the YOU OF NOW...by recognizing the dreams that are living inside you. Spend the majority of your time in the first column...shine a light on the talents, skills and the things you love to do! Allow yourself to savor just the fun things in your life...

OK – Here are the 3 Magic Questions for this exercise:

1. What are the things you are good at? What are things that come naturally to you?
2. What would you do if money didn't matter? If you could quit your job today and dedicate your life to one dream, what would it be?
3. What are the causes that matter most to you? It could be a non-profit, club, social or religious group, political or social cause.

So, what do you love to do? What do you do to give back to the planet? What is your "thing?" Are you a teacher, a healer, a volunteer? Are you a knitter, a stamp collector or a gardener? Do you love to "people watch" or take random rides to places that you've never been? Do you love the fragrance of a flower or doing your family ancestry? Do you love playing the banjo, or taking random pictures of your dog?

Use this list or your journal if you are more comfortable writing this out as a journaling exercise.

So much fun to explore! Let us begin!

THINGS I'M GOOD AT (DO WITH LOVE)
1.
2.
3.
4.
5.
6.
7.
8.
9.
10.
11.
12.
13.
14.
15.
16.
17.
18.
19.
20.

Funny thing...of all of the exercises I give my life-mappers, as excited as they are about thinking about their talents...many get tripped up at putting a label what they are really good at. If this is happening to you, I suggest taking a step back and thinking about the things **other people may tell you that you are good at.** Or just starting with the littler things that bring you joy.

Let's take Marie for example. She also struggled initially to acknowledge her own skills and talents. So, here's how we dug in...

We broke things down into:

1. Things she likes doing for her family and friends
2. Things she likes doing for work/community
3. Things she likes doing for herself

Here's her list:

**THINGS
I'M GOOD AT
(DO WITH LOVE)**

MARIE'S LIST

Family and Friends
1. I'm good at throwing great dinner parties
2. I love finding new recipes to try for my family
3. I'm good at getting to know neighbors
4. I'm good at giving meaningful advice
5. I am a good planner and organizer
6. I love my relationships with other Moms
7. I am good at managing our family finances

Work and Community
1. I'm good at organizing events
2. I'm good at understanding business contracts
3. I care about preserving our towns history
4. I am good at negotiating different ideas and points of view
5. I love town gatherings and the feeling of community
6. I enjoy town politics
7. I love to help people buy and sell homes

Personal
1. I'm a good home decorator
2. I love taking long walks with my dogs on the beach
3. I love to organize our home décor
4. I love investigating my family history

Look carefully at Marie's answers. Do you see how they tell a story? Clearly what came to the surface was her interest in her community service, organizing events and her joy of serving people. As Marie looked at her answers, she was also surprised at how often she listed interests in doing things outside of her day-to-day family responsibilities. This made sense, as her daughters were now off to college, and Marie finally had time to think about therext chapter of life and the contribution she could make outside of her home.

Taking a Tally of Your Talents

Take a look at your lists now...what kind of story does it tell you? Are their things that call out to you? Are there things on your list that you forgot you loved to do? What are the things that fill you, that you do in your spare time or wish you could give more time or attention to? Put a star next to the ones that stand out. We will come back to this special list later.

Designer Dreams in the Now

OK – on to my favorite Lifemapping, life-MAKING exercise of all. Here we you going to design your dream applying Eckart Tolle's Power of the Now. Here you will write out your dream as if you are already living it.

Here is the process:

- **Step One:** You can use your journal for this exercise, or the form below. But for this round, I ask that you set your timer for 10 minutes for your time travel ride into your dream space.

- **Step Two**: Close your eyes and visualize what a moment in your reimagined daily life looks like, using your special skills and talents with the people and places that fill you with love. Think of this as an Instagram snapshot that you are sharing with friends, or a short video clip that provides just a 30 second glimpse of your surroundings. Project yourself into that window and trust the vision that you see.

- **Step Three**: Write the description as if it is happening right now. Let what comes to you, bubble up naturally from the roots of your soul. It can be a few sentences but make it as descriptive as you can. There are no limits here…. you can go anywhere you want, be anything you want, do anything you want…. but make it a vision of you that is filled with peace, contentment, joy and fulfillment.

Let the movie play out in your mind knowing it's coming from a place that you know beyond a shadow of a doubt it is a place that is true for you. There are no limits to what you can do, be achieve, or have.

Have fun on this journey…. Let your dreams fly!

LIVING MY DREAM

Write out your vision of a day or a moment in your best life. What would you be doing if money didn't matter regardless of your current skillset or age? Be as detailed as you can, and write it in present tense, as if you are already living the life of your dreams.

Marie's New Vision

Marie, being the brazen and brawny Jersey girl that she is, was skeptical of this exercise. She'd already tried the vision board, the positive thinking exercises, the mediative affirmations. She was open to all of it of course but said that her brain had a hard time letting her go on this magic carpet ride.

Allowing herself just 10 dedicated minutes of daydreaming, however, after coming off of her talent assessment, put her in an energetically positive space allowing her to invite just a tiny glimpse of what her purpose-connected life could look like. This is what she wrote:

LIVING MY DREAM

Write out your vision of a day or a moment in your best life. What would you be doing if money didn't matter regardless of your current skillset or age? Be as detailed as you can, and write it in present tense, as if you are already living the life of your dreams.

It is early morning and I'm out on the beach walking my dog, talking with a dear friend about the work I'm doing. I've been elected to the town council and there's so much to do...but I am energized. I have so many ideas of things that can be done to make our town even better. People are so appreciative of how I'm contributing and are eager to help support me.

I am both relaxed and excited. The stress I used to feel in my real estate job is gone. I'm still an agent, but the market is so good now, I only need to sell 2-3 houses a year to maintain the income that I need. That leaves me with more than enough time to do my work on the counsel, and still be able to do the things around the house that I love...

My friend and I are planning a dinner party together, to say things to the special friends who have helped get me elected. I'm so grateful to live in a community where I am so close to my neighbors and know that I've created these relationships from a place of mutual trust and respect.

I am fulfilling my inner purpose of giving from myself to my community and the people I care so much about.

Notice the "I am" statements that Marie has put into her vision statement. And, that much of it is "actualizing" the talents and things that she loves to do from her previous exercise. When she shared it with the class, she had a look of contentment on her face. "It actually feels real to me," she said. "It's easy to visualize me walking that beach, having that conversation, so if feels like something that could actually happen."

Less than a year later, Marie was living *that* vision. She had been elected as the town's mayor and her real estate properties were among the highest valued in town. I had the chance to attend a special event that was sponsored by the former city mayor, honoring Marie's contributions to the town that included her receiving a plaque with the "keys to the city." It was a testimony to Marie's hard work, but also how she honored her vision for how to fully transfer her inner purpose to her outer world.

That's what I'd call more than "good enough," Marie. And so, it can be for you.

How to Manifest Your Own Marathon

What was the thing that made Shiz stop by and offer me the opportunity to run the marathon that day? There were certainly other people who she could have asked... colleagues she knew better, who would have been more fit to run that big race. But she came to me. When I look back on it, and where my emotional scale was when she came by, I was in a place of "relaxed openness." I wasn't overly focused on any goal or specific outcome; I was at that time in a state of "being," and just living in the moment. Without requirement or expectation. I wasn't trying to force things to fit any particular agenda. I was in that state of pure allowing.

I found that "power of the now" to be another one of the magical keys of manifestation. The key is to get your vibration to a place of easy openness – not expectation. If I look back to that moment now, I was really just "looking" but not "wanting" – I was calmly open, not overly directed.

And I had also done one really big thing. I asked the universe for help and then I let go.

I think that's what brings it in. You are not blocking with restrictive lists of what the boyfriend should look like or what the job should pay, or when the illness should be cured.

You let go and let God, and you surrender.

Where Is Your Marathon?

While running a marathon was not one of the things that I wanted to do with my life, it too was an exercise that freed me to look at who I was and what I could accomplish in a completely different way.

Within a month after getting back from Boston, I began revaluating everything I had learned from my milestones and my soul guides. I began to dream *really* big and own up to what I really knew in my heart I was here to do. Within a few weeks, I was at a conference and had the opportunity to meet Wayne Dyer in person. I boldly told him about the dream I had and my vision for the impact I wanted to have on the world. I remember my knees shaking as I stood in front of this wonderful man who had written the books that had inspired me most.

With a twinkle in his eye he said, "if you have seen it, it is on its way to you."

And that's where my journey to Discovery began.

SOUL GOODY BAG

Here are some resources mentioned in this chapter for you for further exploration:

- **The Power of Now by Eckhart Tolle** - Much more than simple principles and platitudes, this book takes readers on an inspiring spiritual journey to find their true and deepest self and reach the ultimate goals in personal growth and spirituality: the discovery of truth and light.

- **A New Earth – Awakening to Your Life's Purpose – by Eckhart Tolle** - Tolle shows how transcending our ego-based state of consciousness is not only essential to personal happiness, but also the key to ending conflict and suffering throughout the world.

- **Allison Feehan** - integrativehealingandwellness.com -Allison Feehan is the founder of Integrative Healing and Wellness located in Bay Head, NJ. Trained as a Doctor of Naturopathy with areas of focus around Iridology and Homeopathy, as well as a Reiki Master Teacher, Allison founded the center to provide holistic wellness services to clients. Her work includes individual consultation in the areas of Intuitive Therapy, Reiki, Emotional Freedom Technique, nutrition, meditation, and other innovative Eastern and Western medicines.

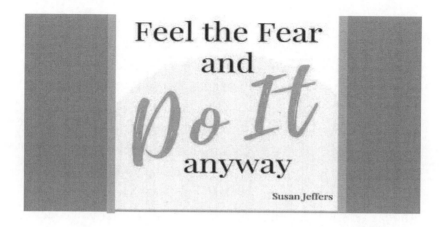

Feel the Fear
and
Do It
anyway

Susan Jeffers

CHAPTER 9

UNVEILING YOUR STORY: THE MEANING IN YOUR MAP

Back in the early eighties, a young entrepreneur named John Hendricks had a big idea. He was a huge fan of documentaries and had a dream of launching a national cable network that would curate and broadcast the best non-fiction films and documentaries. "I was waiting for someone to create my favorite kind of TV channel, Henricks would later write in his biography, and back then nobody was creating it."

John admitted that at the time, he knew relatively little about the TV business, but it was a dream that he couldn't let go of. He went to work, researching every aspect of his big idea and created a business pitch, but the concept was shot down numerous times. Finally, he was able to scrape up enough funding to launch a tiny business. With anxious investors looking over his shoulder, the success of John's dream teetered in the balance, as he faced both financial and personal ruin. But he refused to quit, despite the naysayers, and overwhelming odds against him.

Today, the Discovery Channel is a multi-million dollar global network and parent company to the brands of 19 other channels including HGTV, TLC, Food Network, Animal Planet, Science channel and the Oprah Winfrey Network that are dedication to storytelling that inspires people around the world.

If He Can Do It Why Can't I?

I was reading Henrich's life story "A Curious Discovery," when my plane took off in August 2013, from Dallas to Washington DC. I was on a similar quest. I had used the momentum from my marathon run to launch a vision of my own and John Hendrich's was partly responsible.

It was a time when the world was just beginning to wake up. Authors like Eckhart Tolle, Deepak Chopra and Marianne Williamson were gaining ground as trusted leaders in the soul seeker space. These enlightened teachers were writing books and keynoting sold out teaching expos that were taking the world by storm. And the media was watching, tracking the impact of this new age, mindful movement across the United States and beyond. Then Oprah stepped in offering a chair and a microphone to these "new age authors" that begin on her talk show, and then her network OWN, that was launched by the Discovery Channel and John Hendricks.

In the beginning, OWN was struggling to find its programming footing as well as an audience. I watched with love and fascination, when Oprah launched Super Soul Sunday, and her first Spiritual series, "Belief." But as I waited for more "soulful" content to evolve at OWN, there seemed to be a lull and then a dissipation of this content. I was so disappointed. How could the world not want more of this kind of conversation? There was so much to talk about! So much ancient wisdom to explore. I started making mental notes of all of the shows, series and specials that could come from such a network. Shows about astrology, the afterlife, angels, Atlantis, aromatherapy...and those were just the "A's"!!

That's when my big idea came to me. It was like a lightning bolt that hit me out of nowhere. If Discovery and Oprah had a baby...if it could bring the best of science and curiosity then couple it with Oprah's soulful spirituality, surely, this would create the channel of my dreams!

It would feature stories about seekers who were diving deep into the ancient practices of meditation, and chakra healing and exploration of their past lives. It would tell stories of seekers like me who were looking for purpose and inspiration ... who were thirsting for tools to nourish and replenish their minds, bodies and their spirits. Like Henrich's vision for Discovery, this was a channel that nobody was creating. So, it was time to take my dream to Discovery.

Wait, what? Who me? Come on.... what was I thinking?

But the idea took hold of me... I became obsessed with thinking about it.

When I sat down and wrote out the vision for my big idea, it seemed utterly crazy on paper. The decision required me to face a lot of fear. Here's a very partial list of what my ego dictated to me:

1. You have no experience starting a network.

2. You would be leaving behind a lucrative paycheck and job security at the company that has supported and promoted you.

3. You would be uprooting your entire family (again) to another brand-new state (and Texas was a disaster, remember?)

4. You are no spring chicken, in fact, you are 50 years old.

5. No one has done this so far and, if it was such a great idea, someone a lot smarter than you would have already done it.

All true...all true.

But here's the thing...when the voice of inspiration speaks...it is not a voice at all...it's a yearning you feel inside of you. You can't let go of it...and it won't let go of you.

But this time, I threw aside the voice of my ego... and gave my heart a chance to speak. Here's what my sweet little heart reminded me, regarding those above statements:

1. You have a ton of experience working in TV and helped AT&T start their TV business. John Hendricks didn't either. You are an award-winning producer.

2. You mean leaving the company that pays you for the job where your soul is dying?

3. Your family hates Texas. They are ready for the next adventure.

4. You just ran the fucking Boston Marathon thank you very much.

5. Every single person you share this idea with, loves it.

In the end, I think my heart pitched a better argument. So, what did I do? **I felt the fear and did it anyway**. I held the vision. **I took action.**

Four months later, I was in my new office at Discovery, ready to launch my dream.

And it can be the same for you.

Bringing Your Story to Life

You have done so much of your soul work already...and this next chapter will bring your lifemap into view. And as with any map, it can be a tad overwhelming if you just try to take in all of the detail, without an intention of where you are going... so here's how we are going to approach that goal so the next two chapters will be about being on the road, versus getting on the road. So, shall we?

In this chapter we will....

- **Ego-test Your Day Dream** – We'll take the "Best Day" exercise from the last chapter and bench-test it against your fears. This will help us shake out any doubts, objections, or measures of "not enough-ness" that could cloud your vision and cause any roadblocks on your route ahead.

- **Unveil Your Lifemapping Story -** Yes, THIS IS IT! Here's where we will overlay all of your "I am's," into one cohesive view of the amazing, meaningful, bountiful you. This is where you'll bring together all of your love and fear lessons to really see the story that has become your foundation. Then you will use it as a springboard for creating the path forward to the life of your purpose.

- **Identify and Release**- This is where I'll help you with tools and tricks for mentally moving those fear-based roadblocks that will help repave your way forward. This is where you will learn how to identify and silence that inner chatter that interferes with your now... disarming those thoughts, beliefs and limited ideas that have kept you from making the choices and decisions for you to grow on purpose.

No More Would-A, Could-A, Should-A's.

This is where your life review, becomes your life *renew*... where you get to see the beautiful, self-actualized, self-orchestrated map of your soul. This is where you can step back and begin to see the tapestry of your life and how those threads have woven the fabric of who you are, and what you have come to offer the world. Feel the Fear and Do It anyway...will help you with ideas and exercises for releasing the fear and setting the intentions for your lifetime from here.

This sounds hard. And it kind of is. I won't lie to you. It took a lot of work to get me from Dallas to Discovery.

But here's the thing that I kept saying to myself that kept me motivated, and it boiled down to these three powerful words- Rocking Chair Remorse.

It was the vision I had of the future me...the "old woman me" sitting in a rocking chair somewhere. Reflecting on my life. Re-reviewing all those dang yellow sticky notes on the wall. How would I feel? What stories would I be telling? Would it be savory or sour? Would it be a tale of acquiescing or adventure? I could see that women with the wrinkles and wiry grey hair in my mind's eye winking at me. It was like we were making a deal with each other from the future, and I didn't want to let the "future" me down.

So, I went back to my Lifemapping exercise one more time. I decided what I needed to do was gather all of those lessons I had uncovered together and stick them back up on my wall one more time. I took my milestones, and my soul squad, about what I was and wasn't good at and put it all up there – in one place. They sat displayed ... NAKED & AFRAID, so I could shine a light on it all and figure out how to activate my dream. To *really* ponder what my heart was yearning for. Truth be told, a small part of me just wanted to see if any of this Lifemapping shit worked...at all.

I'll show you the full view in a moment. But before we get there there's one last exercise that I'd like you to do to round out the full picture of your map.

How to Ego Test Your Daydream

So, at the end of the last chapter, Marie wrote out her beautiful picture of a beautiful life moment, where she could see her walking blissfully along the seaside with her friend, talking about how she had fulfilled her dream. Using her list of the things she loved to do, she was able to ride that wave of positive energy vibration right into her vision of the perfect day.

It was the perfect way to end the chapter on "Embracing our Purpose"

But how do we hold fast to that perfect vision and positive energy when the fear monger steps in? That same voice that came to throw cold water on me when I jumped into my big dream of going to Discovery. In other words, how do you tell your ego to "shut up!?"

You will need some powerful combat weapons for this my friend, which I promise, you will receive once we get through this next exercise. And since we're now in the "Feel the Fear and Do It Anyway" Zone, we're going to call out our EGOs from their place in the shadows and nail them to their own list. In other words, we are call them out for the imposters that they are and get them off our manifestation highway!

You up for some gunslinging here? Trust me...it'll be gritty, but in a good way. Like flossing.

Go Ahead, Make My Day

I love that expression from that old Clint Eastwood movie... that vision of him taking aim at the bad guy daring them to do their worst because he's armed, with his finger on the trigger, aiming his powerful weapon at them, ready to take them out.

And so, it is with this next exercise. You are going to place your aim at all those trickster sabotages to your perfect day, and you are going to call them out for the nasty liars and imposters that they are so you can tick them off with your weapon of truth, one by one, like target practice in a shooting gallery.

C'mon...BE the Clint. Let's do this.

LIFEMAP EXPLORATION #8 — Part 1

Unveiling
Your Story
(Part 1)

With this exercise we are going to get right into it. This is where we "Life Proof Your Vision." We are going to look these ego-driven excuses right in the eye and take them to task. No softie soul-affirmations just yet. Not until we get these cleared out of Dodge.

Step One: Revisit Your Vision: Go back to Chapter 8 on pg ## and re-read your "Living Your Dream" day. Breathe in how good it feels. Really be there for a moment. You feel it? You believe it, right? You know, beyond a shadow of a doubt, that it's coming to you...that it **will be** your future.

Wait...what was that? Did you feel it? That "Bloop?" It might pop up like a little ping around your solar plexus... or just a slight hint of heaviness that crops up in the back of your mind...behind your ear perhaps. It might feel like a little nervous flicker...a little pause... a dip of your energy. That my friend, your infiltrator, is also known as "doubt."

Doubt has no place in your perfect day. Doubt must be eliminated. So, this is where you are going to write up the list of things that challenge you from doing what you love. We are going to call those naysayers out!

Step Two: ID the Perpetrators: Infiltrators like doubt are the thoughts that come in to tell you why "logically speaking," your dream will most likely not come true. After that, the terrible word "but..." can creep in, followed very quickly (if you don't stop it) by the justification for *why* your vision could actually not come true. You've grown up with these justifiers. "But's" best compadre is "not enough." As in- "I have a big, beautiful house..." (then the "doubt bloop" happens) and you finish your sentence with the words, "....**but not enough** money." Similarly, perhaps you think to yourself, *"I have an amazing job...* **but** *I don't have* **enough** *experience to land my dream job."* What are you biggest challenging statements preventing you from doing what you love?

With any affirmation of the future, there is always the danger of the doubt bloop creeping in. But fear not. This is the place where we will point our gun at those little mental termites so you can prevent them from gnawing away at your vision.

Step Three: Use the list below to write out and tally up the nay-sayers. Write everything that comes to you just as they drum up every excuse for why your dream can't happen. And then get ready to say those powerful words, "Go ahead, make my day." Remind them who has the power here!

Don't worry... we are going to put all of those perpetrators under arrest.

Oh, and for reference, here's my list of "doubt bloops" – may they rest in peace.

THINGS THAT CHALLENGE OR PREVENT ME FROM DOING WHAT I LOVE
1. I don't have enough time
2. I don't have enough experience
3. It will be too hard on my family
4. It's a financial risk
5. I could fail
6. I don't have enough self-confidence
7. I might not be strong enough
8. I might not have enough talent
9. I'm afraid of being judged
10. I'm afraid what people will think
11. I don't have the right resume
12. I might be too old
13. I would have to start over
14. I don't have enough help
15. It will be too much work
16. Not enough people believe in it/me.

THINGS THAT CHALLENGE OR PREVENT ME FROM DOING WHAT I LOVE
1.
2.
3.
4.
5.
6.
7.
8.
9.
10.
11.
12.
13.
14.
15.
16.
17.
18.
19.
20.

Ah...I can feel you from here...this list looks pretty, well... convincing right? Each and every one of those reasons, the "not enough's," the "might's" and the "might nots" are all just sending out their words of warning. They are wanting to protect you... keep you in your comfort zone, safe from a mis-step and from losing everything you've already worked so hard for. They don't want you to be exposed as the "less than" you might be.

But stop...right...there!! That voice IS NOT YOU!! That is the voice of EGO. That is the voice of FEAR. They are going to try to talk you out of the thing that you came here to do.

But you have the power to turn your back on it and stay in your truth. And before this chapter is over, you will know how.

Fear and Finding the Self Within

Sometimes, we are called to question everything we've been taught that was right and responsible, when life sends us a curve ball, challenging everything we know and have come to believe. I have found that those who are given some of the most insurmountable challenges are the ones that are given the biggest opportunities to make their hardest choices. It's that fork in the road that presents itself... and yup, you guessed it, it's the choice between the right onto Love Lane or the left onto Fear Freeway.

It is in those moments when it seems the most logical and justified to play it safe. Ah but those with the greatest stories are the ones that chose to take that road less traveled. And that has made all the difference in their lives. One of those heroes is my friend and fellow lifemapper Sheila.

Hers is a story of overcoming, transforming, re-emerging and flourishing.

SHEILA'S STORY: Singing from a New Sheet of Music

If you'd met Sheila three years ago, you wouldn't have recognized her. Vibrant, beautiful, quick witted, and full of life, she has literally metamorphized before my very eyes.

When we first met, Sheila was SVP of the largest advertising agencies in the country. She was giving a presentation in our corporate board room that included our top executives. It was a pitch that, if successful, would land her firm a ten-million-dollar account in the first year.

Sheila was an expert show woman who infused every idea with a perfectly played combo of magnetic charm and sarcasm. She was so enthusiastic and warmly passionate, there was no way you could resist wanting to work with her.

A few weeks into our new project, Sheila and I became fast friends on our daily conference calls. Things were off to a strong start, and I was thrilled at the progress we were making together. One morning, I received the devasting news that Sheila's husband had died very suddenly. There were few details, but I was told that he had a heart attack.

"I'm not sure when she'll be back to work." they told me. There were no words. I knew that Sheila didn't have children, but I had no insight on her family or support system. I sent her a note, offering her any support I could.

I was shocked when Sheila was back in the office, three days later. After getting through my condolences, I quietly asked her if she thought she was ready to be back in the office so soon. "Absolutely," she responded. "Really, I'm fine. It's better for me to work...and there's so much to do!"

And so, as it always does with corporate America, work life carried on. Two months later, the first draft of our project proposal was submitted and approved. I set up a congratulatory phone call for the entire team to celebrate, but Sheila didn't show.

Three days went by without word from her. Alarmed, I called another colleague at her agency. Sheila had ended up in the emergency room. The reasons weren't known.

When Sheila came back to the office, her entire demeanor had changed. Her enthusiasm had waned, and she was quiet during meetings. I tried multiple times to reach out to her, but she avoided any conversation about her wellness. It was as if a light that had switched off inside of her. Time marched on...and hard as I tried, I could not break through the shield that she had put up between us.

Fast forward four years later when I got a call from Sheila who I hadn't seen in ages. "Karen, do you have time to catch up?"

Our conversation revealed a side of Sheila that I didn't know. A tumultuous journey through an adoptive childhood. An abusive husband, who was a heavy drinker and drug-user. Her own alcohol problem that she had been hiding for years. A marriage that had been a failed substitute for love. And a career that had been a mask to hide years of her insecurity and shame.

"When he died, it triggered so much guilt and failure that I felt within myself that I didn't even know was there. I woke up one morning and realized that my entire life has been a cover up."

Sheila was ready to start over. She had successfully completed a year of sobriety, but wasn't finding success with traditional psychotherapy. I told her about my Lifemapping exercise.

"Oh my gosh...that's what I have to do. Can you show me?"

THINGS THAT CHALLENGE OR PREVENT ME FROM DOING WHAT I LOVE
Sheila's List

1. I can't sing
2. Well, I can't sing well
3. I have no musical training
4. Well, I took piano lessons for 3 months before I quit
5. I never took voice lessons
6. I don't like being told what to do
7. I'm afraid to give up my safe job
8. I am my own sole breadwinner
9. The odds of my success is low
10. The odds of making money doing this is low
11. I won't be able to live alone in NYC and afford an apartment
12. I could really fail. Like in a really big way
13. People might hate my singing
14. If I fail, I might start drinking again
15. Oh, and did I mention, I am old. Who does something like this when they are 55?

Going through her milestones helped Sheila understand how her adoptive childhood made her so fiercely independent and strong. "I felt like I had to market myself to my parents every day, so they wouldn't send me back," she said. "The feeling of being abandoned by my natural parents was always there... it was a feeling of not being good enough. I know I carried that through into my marriage and he felt that. We both just numbed ourselves from the pain of not getting the love we both needed."

What surprised me the most was Sheila's feelings about her career. Her success, she said, came from the need to control the outcome of her life, but it was never her true calling, and covered up a lifetime of longing to be on stage, and share her songs as an entertainer.

Turning Sheila's Pain into Her Passion

It was easy for Sheila to write out her vision of her perfect day, visualizing herself in a small cabaret theatre, smiling and interacting with her audience, seated behind her piano. But her list of "Things Preventing Me from Doing What I Love" was what she wanted to focus on. After going through her list, she understood that the majority of her fears, were based on her innate lack of "enough-ness" that started at birth. Now it was about having the courage to leave that behind her.

By all counts, it was a daunting list.

Is it possible to take a huge vision like Sheila's and truly make it a dream come true?

Yep. One hundred percent.

In the next Chapter, we're going to learn how to take your list, as well as the unfolded vision of your lifemap to re-craft your thoughts and words to create the vision you've dreamed of so that you feel it energetically and emotionally. As we learned from Eckart in the last chapter, the feeling attached to the belief and how you feel about it in the "now," is key to manifesting the vision itself.

For now, I'll let you in on where Sheila is today. She's completed her first critically acclaimed one woman show in New York City, and has started a new life with a new partner, (who also happens to be her voice coach and piano instructor). Her current relationship is bringing her the love, validation and connection that she's always dreamed of. In her words, "I've gotten more than the dream, I've gotten the reality."

And not one of those items on her list has power over her any longer.

Way to go Sheila!

Bringing Your Lifemap into View

As you bring all of the people, places and events of your life in one place, it will begin to tell a story. It's like stitching together a patchwork quilt that initially looks like it is a checkerboard of unrelated materials, until it is displayed in one cohesive view.

In this case, the magic is in the juxtaposition of love placed with its opposite, fear, for you to see first-hand. I've included mine on the next page, to show you what it will look like when it's finished.

This will show you the DNA of your soul. You will be surprised by how love and fear have been working together, hand and hand, all along ... for your entire life- FOR YOU.

Wanna see? (It's really magical... I'm so excited for you!)

Let's just do a quick soul-firmation here, since this is such a big moment. Let's breathe in all of the possibilities that are to come!

 SOULFIRMATION #9

"I marvel
at all I have accomplished
and how it shines a light on my path.
I am right on track.
I see my life in a whole new way."

LIFEMAPPING EXPLORATION #8: Part 2

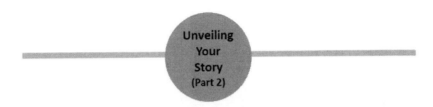

To get this vision started, let's begin by taking a look at my compiled list on the next page.

Don't let all of that information scare you. Trust me, it looks more complicated than it is in practice. This is like compiling a patch work quilt. It is simply transferring the information that you have compiled about your life in the previous steps and putting it in one place. And this, IS where your lifemap will show your life's purpose.

Putting Your Map Together

OK this Is how we do it ... it's a cut and paste job.

There is a blank template on the next page in case you want to follow my format. You can also just print them out and tape them on your wall like I initially did.

OK, here we go.

- **Step #1 – Grab Your "Life Milestones"** - Go back to Chapter 6 (p.##) to your "Things I Learned About Myself From My Major LOVE Milestones" and "Things I learned about Myself from My Fear Milestones." Transfer those lists to Column #1 and #2.

- **Step #2 – Grab Your "Soul Squad Lessons"** - Go back to Chapter 7 (p. ##) to your "Things I Learned From my Fear Squad" and "Things I learned from my Love Squad." Add those lists to Column #3 and #4

- **Step #3 – Grab Your "Good At's"** - Go back to Chapter 8 (p.##) and add the "I'm Good At" list to Column #5.

- **Step #4 – Grab Your "Challenge Me's"** – Go back to the beginning of this chapter. Add the "Challenge Me's" to Column #6.

Feel free to use this template below and I've shared my own Key Takeaways Exploration on p. 257, just because we are on this journey together!

MY LIFE MAP: Key Takeaways

THINGS I LEARNED FROM MY LOVE MILESTONES	THINGS I LEARNED FROM MY FEAR MILESTONES	THINGS I LEARNED FROM MY LOVE SQUAD	THINGS I LEARNED FROM MY FEAR SQUAD	THINGS I'M GOOD AT (DO WITH LOVE)	THINGS THAT CHALLENGE or PREVENT ME FROM DOING WHAT I LOVE
1.–20.	1.–20.	1.–20.	1.–20.	1.–20.	1.–20.
What I Need to Teach	What I Need to Learn	Who I Came to Be	What I Came to Overcome	What I Came to Give	What I Came to Release

MY LIFE MAP: Key Takeaways

THINGS I LEARNED FROM MY LOVE MILESTONES	THINGS I LEARNED FROM MY FEAR MILESTONES	THINGS I LEARNED FROM MY LOVE SQUAD	THINGS I LEARNED FROM MY FEAR SQUAD	THINGS I'M GOOD AT (DO WITH LOVE)	THINGS THAT CHALLENGE or PREVENT ME FROM DOING WHAT I LOVE
1. I am strong	1. I am a harsh judge of myself	1. I am a storyteller	1. I am not smart enough	1. I am good at making people happy/feel good about themselves	1. I don't have enough time
2. I am a seeker	2. I am not smart enough	2. I am unconditionally loved	2. I am not talented enough	2. I am good at teaching others about the things that inspire me	2. I don't have enough experience
3. I am spiritual	3. I am not good enough	3. I love unconditionally	3. I am not pretty enough	3. I am good at exploring and sharing spiritual concepts	3. It will be too hard on my family
4. I am smart	4. I am fearful	4. I am a talented writer/storyteller/producer	4. I am not worth loving	4. I am a good writer/producer	4. It's a financial risk
5. I am intuitive	5. I am full of self-doubt	5. I am a mentor/supporter	5. I am insignificant	5. I am good at supporting those I love and care about	5. I could fail
6. I am compassionate	6. I am useless	6. I am creative/creator	6. I am not creative	6. I am good at getting up after I fall down	6. I don't have enough self-confidence
7. I don't give up/am resilient	7. I am not brave	7. I am kind	7. I am not articulate	7. I am good at meditating	7. I might not be strong enough
8. I am caring	8. I am afraid of confrontation	8. I am an uplifter	8. I am not successful	8. I am a good at listening with my heart	8. I might not have enough talent
9. I am courageous	9. I am not confident	9. I am wise	9. I am not worthy of my dream	9. I am good at practicing gratitude	9. I'm afraid of being judged
10. I am always giving my best	10. I am not a good person	10. I am intuitive	10. I am not a good person	10. I am good at allowing my children follow their own path	10. I'm afraid what people will think
11. I am a doer/create big goals	11. I am afraid of being judged	11. I am a teacher	11. I am not committed enough		11. I don't have the right resume
12. I am inspired	12. I am afraid they will see through me	12. I am a achiever	12. I am not strong enough		12. I might be too old
13. I am good at following my instincts	13. I am afraid to fail	13. I am brave	13. I am not worthy of loyalty		13. I would have to start over
14. I am a learner	14. I am too attached to success and outcome	14. I am persistent	14. I am not a good leader		14. I don't have enough help
15. I am an inspirer	15. I am afraid of speaking my truth	15. I am loyal	15. I am a failure		15. It will be too much work
16. I am an explorer	16. I am quick to blame myself	16. I am an inspirational leader	16. I am not brave enough		16. Not enough people believe in it/me.
17. I am a survivor	17. I am too nice	17. I am a visionary	17. I am too nice		
18. I am powerful	18. I am not strong enough	18. I am an innovator	18. I am not paying attention to what's important		
19. I am grateful/appreciative	19. I am different	19. I am a seeker	19. I am selfish		
20. I am an uplifter	20. I am selfish	20. I am believer	20. I am not dependable		
What I Need to Teach	**What I Need to Learn**	**Who I Came to Be**	**What I Came to Overcome**	**What I Came to Give**	**What I Came to Release**

When you have completed your table, take a moment and really take inventory of all of the things that you have written on this page. Reread them. Look at all of the similarities and all of the contradictions. Take a moment and capture some of these takeaways in your journal

- What story emerges of you?
- Take a step back and try to objectively look at this person through divine, non-judgmental eyes...like a mother would look at their child...what emotions come to the surface?
- How do you feel about yourself?
- What didn't you know about yourself before that you see now?
- Do you feel differently?

For me, this picture became a complete catharsis .... a recognition and releasing of so many emotions. Instead of self-judgement, I could see myself as the soul I was... who had come to this planet on a mission... and who was, through earnest intention and vast mistakes, trying to fulfill that contract. In fact, I was taking on both pain and joy with a determination to get it right in order to fulfill that contract!

I felt empathy for me. I felt proud of me. LOL – I wanted to hug me.

I don't know about you, but one of my biggest life's challenges, at its basis, has been trying to find my way to self-love. And finally, with those columns filled out, I was able to see the soul of "me" from behind the façade of me. And on that page of "I am's" I couldn't hide.

This is so powerful my friend...and I recognize it as hard work. This is your life review, and it can also be your life wakeup call...and life reset.

Take a moment to write down in your journal, the thoughts, feelings or insights that you receive as a result of looking at this wholistic and holistic view of you. If it feels right, answer those questions above.

This is such an important portrait of who you are within and without... and it is the map to where we go from here.

I'm so proud of how far you've come!

The Difference Between Being Brave and Being Fearless

When I was getting ready to write this book, the biggest thing standing in my way was fear. Even though I was clear that I wanted to share this concept of Lifemapping, and already had many friends asking me to share my workshops, when it came time to facing the first few chapters, I felt frozen-down to the level of asking the most basic of questions.

Who was I...to even think I had any level of expertise to create this book? Even though I knew the process had worked for me, and for the people who had attended my workshops, I was – wait for it – fearful that I wouldn't have the credibility, to really connect with my reader.

Once again, my ever-diligent publisher-to-be Melanie Warner, was on top of this. She would cheer on our small group of wanna-be writers, who were all in their own way slowly drowning in the overwhelm of uncertainty. As a published author herself, Melanie knew what we were experiencing. Always the energetic preacher of publishing with her Texas accent, she with little fanfare, told us that it was our own selves and nothing else, that was holding us back.

If it weren't for one word, your books would be published by now. Yeah, you guessed it.

"Fear stands for **F**alse **E**vidence **A**ppearing **R**eal." She said. "When you perceive something to be true, you believe it. Anything that is making you stuck and holding you back is because of fear. Whether it is fear of failure, or even fear of success. It is one little word that has so much power over us."

Melanie knew what she was talking about from firsthand experience. Not only as a publisher, and bestselling author. She had buried a child, gone through a divorce, lost her home and business, and had to start her own life over again. A few times.

Melanie boiled the fear outcomes down into what she called "The Three Modalities of Fear" or the things that stop us from trying the things we know in our hearts we should do:

> #1 – If I try, I could **fail**
> #2 – People won't like me, or they will judge me in a **negative way**
> #3 – I'm **not worthy**

Before we were allowed to go any further in the writing of our books, Melanie asked us to look at these three modalities and identify which spoke the loudest to us. She made us carefully evaluate each one and identify which one was the trap we were falling into that was holding us back.

Then she shared they real truth. The mind-blowing thing about each Fear modality is that you are just as likely to have a positive outcome, as a negative one... which coincidently is exactly the same thing that we just demonstrated in our

Lifemapping exercise. Fear has always got a flip side... and it's up to you to decide which team you want to play on..

> #1 – If I try, I could **succeed**
> #2 – People would like me and judge me in a **positive way**.
> #3 – I **am worthy**

This is exactly what we are doing in this book – taking a look at the fear and flipping it on its head and turning the love light on it baby. And IT-IS-POWERFUL!!

Here's the thing... there's always the potential to fail at anything we do. In fact, often, failure is the thing that propels us to success. Sometimes it pisses us off so much we just want to kick it in the ass. And sometimes, it's simply because doing what have to is planted in us like a rocket that is attached to our backs that we can control.

If you feel that fear is holding you back from really owning your dream vision, I get you. I sat for most of my life in the front row pew of that church. But here's the key...most of the time our greatest fears NEVER come to pass. Instead, they just hold us frozen in the moment and keep us from doing the things we know we are here to do. It holds us back from following our intuition...the whisper of our soul.

It can be big things like "I'd love to move to the beach." "I'd love to say hello to that cute guy at Starbucks." "I really want to try skydiving" Do you feel the passion there? The sense of yearning of your heart's desire? That is the whisper of your soul.

Fear-Releasers

Before we can move on from our current place of new awareness and move into the final step of Activating our Lifemap, meaning taking these insights and creating your plan, we need to attend to one really important piece of business. Your FEAR RELEASE. Because no matter what you've learned from this exercise, it will continue to hold you back if you don't take its power away.

Let's be real...fear never goes away. Not really...that last statement is incorrect. Fear is the one thing, that no matter what happens to us, we have the choice to embrace or turn our backs on. But it can be really, really hard to do. Believe me, I know, but there are a few "magic spells" that you can use to help banish Fear from your party. So, let's take a look at a few things you can try if you feel the fear bug creeping back in too close to your soul sandwich.

I like to call on these release exercises to give fear the big "heave ho."

And then, as we sit in that glow of yearning, the shadow of the ego emerges. The voice of the what if...now it's time for our inner Clint Eastwood to do its thing. Let's kick those negative naysayers out the door.

Here are some easy/powerful (my favorite combination) ways of releasing fear, blame and uncertainty. Rather than dictate one specifically for you, I invite you to choose from one the ideas below.

I have done all of them, and each has been a very effective way to release those "doubt bloops" as well as worries, afterthoughts, second-guesses and maybe's.

This may feel slightly silly if you haven't done anything like this before but I promise you, if you give one or more a try, it will help you train your mind that those fearful thoughts are not welcome. Eventually these fearful thoughts will be itemized and banished.

1. **Do a Burning Ceremony** – Write down all of your fears on a piece of paper. Acknowledge the role they have played in your life and then rip the paper up into tiny pieces. Safely light each paper and send the fear off into the Universe.

2. **Rise & Release** -Put all of your fear thoughts into an imaginary basket. You can read them out-loud or simply associate one word to each fear, but one by one...put them mentally together. Imagine yourself tying a huge helium balloon to the basket and letting it go. Watch it rise into the sky.... higher and higher, and finally disappearing out of sight.

3. **Write A Post about your Accomplishment** – Type out a quick 15 sentence post that you can share on social media that tells the world about your accomplishment as if you Have Already Done it. If you have a photo of your vision, add it to your story. In your description explain how you faced your fear and did it anyway.

4. **Forgiveness Releaser** – If remapping your path forward requires releasing feelings of anger, guilt, mistrust or sadness, these emotions will also keep you in a place from manifesting your vision. Take a moment to visualize the person or experience that has hurt you and write them a letter. If you can send a message of forgiveness to that soul or situation, it will free you from the dark emotions of that experience, and allow opportunities of love to fill into that space.

Feel the Fear and Do It Anyway

Feel the Fear and Do it Anyway is an actual book written by Susan Jeffers. She appeared many times on the Oprah show, and was deemed the "queen of self-help" in the early eighties. I consulted her book often, as there weren't many "how-to's" for fear, back when I was graduating from college.

Hers is also a great story of a seeker who walked the walk, and overcame her own self-doubts in getting her book published. In the preface, she tells the story of how it was rejected from so many publishers that she almost gave up. "After all," she wrote, "if you received a rejection letter, as I did, that said, 'Lady Di could be cycling nude down the street giving this book away, nobody would read it,' wouldn't you be tempted to give up trying?"

She went on to say that she actually put the manuscript away in a drawer for a few years and almost forgot about it until one day she rediscovered it, and couldn't push away the feeling that it had something important to say. "So, I made a vow to myself," she said. "Somehow, I am going to find a way to Feel the Fear...and Do It Anyway, and get this book out into the world."

Susan went on to sell millions of copies of her book, and wrote 17 more, sharing tools and wisdom to help people enjoy a deeper, richer and happier life. Susan, like many of those early spiritual gurus seeded the idea that we are all divine souls whose Higher Selves are here to learn on our earthly path.

"I have come to believe that there are only two kinds of experiences in life," she wrote. "Those that stem from our Higher Self and those that have much to teach us. We recognize the first as pure joy and the latter as struggle. But they are both perfect. Each time we confront some intense difficulty, we know there is something that we haven't learned yet and the universe is now giving us an opportunity to learn.... Nothing is as satisfying as those moments of breakthrough when you discover something about yourself and the universe that adds another piece to the jigsaw puzzle. The joy of discovery is delicious. I know of no other explorer who once having reached his or her goal has not wanted to go out and explore some more." P.205

Susan ends her book reposting one of her favorite passages about the loves and the fears that infuse our life's journeys throughout our walk here. This passage is one of my favorites too. It's from the Velveteen Rabbit by Margery Williams. In the story, two nursery toys, the Skin Horse and the Rabbit, talk about becoming real.

> *"Real isn't how you are made,' said the Skin Horse. 'It's a thing that happens to you. When a child loves you for a long, long time, not just to play with, but REALLY loves you, then you become Real.*
>
> *'Does it hurt?' asked the Rabbit.*
>
> *'Sometimes,' said the Skin Horse, for he was always truthful. 'When you are Real you don't mind being hurt.'*
>
> *'Does it happen all at once, like being wound up,' he asked, 'or bit by bit?'*
>
> *'It doesn't happen all at once,' said the Skin Horse. 'You become. It takes a long time. That's why it doesn't happen often to people who break easily, or have sharp edges, or who have to be carefully kept. Generally, by*

the time you are Real, most of your hair has been loved off, and your eyes drop out and you get loose in the joints and very shabby. But these things don't matter at all, because once you are Real you can't be ugly, except to people who don't understand.'"

—Margery Williams Bianco, The Velveteen Rabbit

It is all about the joy of your own self-discovery. Susan Jeffries knew it and dared herself to publish her book. John Hendricks knew it and dared to create a global network based on curiosity and discovery. And you will do it too.

SOUL GOODY BAG

Here are some resources mentioned in this chapter for you for further exploration:

- **A Curious Discovery by John Hendricks** - John Hendricks shares the remarkable story of building one of the most successful media empires in the world, Discovery Communications and reveals that his professional achievements would not have been possible without one crucial quality that has informed his life since childhood: curiosity.

- **Feel the Fear and Do It Anyway by Dr. Susan Jeffers.** Whatever your fear, here is your chance to push through it once and for all. In this enduring guide to self-empowerment, Dr. Susan Jeffers inspires us with dynamic techniques and profound concepts that have helped countless people grab hold of their fears and move forward with their lives.

SECTION THREE

WHERE YOU ARE HEADED: YOUR LIFEMAPPING PATH FORWARD...

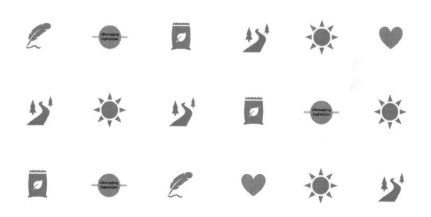

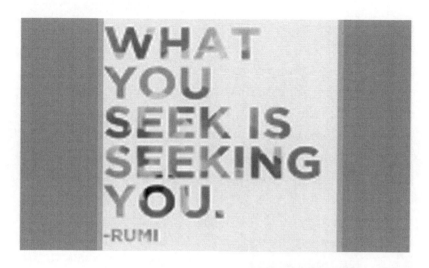

WHAT YOU SEEK IS SEEKING YOU.
-RUMI

CHAPTER 10

ACTIVATING YOUR LIFEMAP

And then, just when you think you've got it all figured out... it happens.

One minute you're in control.... riding high...cruising carefree down the manifestation super-highway. You've got the top down, the wind at your back, and the sun is just peeking out from the horizon rising on a blissful new day. You've got your fears at bay...your ego in check, your higher self is secure at the wheel, driving off towards destiny. You are, as Abraham Hicks would often say, "tuned in, tapped in, turned on."

And then... you hit a pothole. Your tire blows out. You total the entire car. Suddenly, you are stuck out there in the middle of the desert wondering how it happened and what in tarnation, you're supposed to do next.

Has that ever happened to you?

I have to be honest. As much as I would love to be that person who "lived eternally in the fearless zone, in the now… wearing my lavender oil infused frock, in an ever-present moment of allowing-ness," the truth is, at the root of me, I was none of those things. There has always been this driven (like a Mack-truck, mother-load of "I'm going to freaking make this happen, GDMit") part of me that has compelled me through most my entire life. It's the, "Hey if I don't do this, it won't get done, right?" need for controlling things to assure that it delivers my exact intended and desired expectations. Sound familiar?

So why is it that when our car breaks down, or veers of the road, it shakes things up so much for us?

Hint? It's all about the control baby.

Science fiction novelist, Kurt Vonnegut Jr, once coined the phrase, "I am a human being, not a human doing." I loved the sarcastic turn of that statement…the rebellious bent aimed against that daily grind of doing. But there I was at a loss. I just didn't know how to **do** that be-ing thing. I mean how could that get anyone, anywhere?

My credo, has always been about the DO-ing. I gotta make lists, I MUST have an action plan. I gotta **do stuff to make stuff** happen.

That's my "manifest-o…"

That's how it works, right?

Oh, was I ever going to learn how wrong that was! It was time for the Universe to step in and set me straight because, in my humanness, I had forgotten.

The trick really a pretty simple:

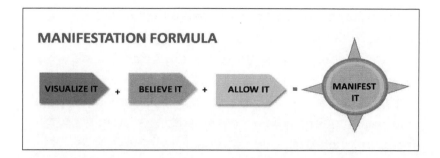

That's the formula for manifestation. (I would highlight that if I were you because we'll come back to this.)

Oh but there is still so much still to share with you!

In this chapter we will:

- **Tally your Takeaway's:** This is where the magic happens...where your map reveals its story...this is where we take the incredible work that you did in the last chapter of laying out your lifemap and here we simplify the story to show you what you came to learn and what you came to do.

  Here is where you will select 3 Key "I am" statements that you feel ring truest for you and bounce up the strongest vibrations on your love and fear scale. These are the beckoning's of your life's purpose.

- **Learn the Manifestation Formula:** Yes, there is a real magic spell to making your dreams come true! I'll explain the 4-step process that took my vision from idea to fruition, and help you identify places that might be tripping you up on your own manifestation journey.

This chapter is where you will begin to build on your map by taking everything in your love column and amplifying it. And flipping anything in the fear side to the positive, so it doesn't have any more power over you. This is the part where you map your story *on purpose*...to YOUR purpose for your lifetime.

This magic will shine through in your "I am's... the sparkly soul-full uniqueness of you. And stating, owning, emitting and energizing the power of you.

The manifestation formula IS about the doing, but it's also about the being and allowing. They work together as a team.

Let me explain how I figured that out.

A Funny Thing Happened when I got to Discovery.

I thought I had everything all figured out when I visualized my way into that "dream job." And it was a dream job... I have envisioned it and manifested it. It was such a great story to tell! I mean I really knew how to visualize and materialize. Heck, even I was inspired by me! But it didn't go at all as I expected. Not one iota.

Let me back up, and tell you how I got there. When I made up my mind that I wanted to do that Discovery job I was able to truly get myself to a place where I was aligned with that vision. I just KNEW that was where I needed to be and that all my life experience had led me to be there... to bring this idea to life. I – JUST – KNEW – IT.

And then, as the universe does, it goes out of its way to bring your vision to you. "Ask and it is Given." And it all just came to me like magic.

It started with me verbalizing my dream out loud.

So, I talked to my friend Kurt. Kurt was someone who "saw me..." Kurt was a high performing "do-er" on our team. He and his partner had recently adopted a baby girl, and his vison of the world was softening. We'd just left one of our soul-sucking meetings, and were commiserating about what we'd do if we could ever be freed from our corporate prison cells. When I told him about my "Oprah and Discovery" vision, his eyes lit up.

"Oh girl," he said, "Does your universe EVER love you!"

As it turned out, the head of Discovery's Creative Services group was his dear friend and former college roommate. Kurt connected us. We set up a phone meeting. We hit it off. I got an interview. And then, BOOM! Within three months, I not only got the job, they created a new role specifically FOR ME! On January 5, 2015, I checked into my bright yellow office in Discovery's Silver Spring Maryland Headquarters.

Abracadabra baby...

And so good... good for me. It was a big deal. I had left my family behind in Dallas to put the house on the market. I moved into a tiny little apartment a two block walk from work. It was my mid-life moment...I was taking action! I was following my bliss! I was on my way to Discovery.

And then, that's when my manifestation took a little shifty....

You can't always get what you want (but if you try, sometimes you get what you need).

Have you ever had one of those dreams where you were running and suddenly your legs fell like they weighed a thousand pounds and you are trying to move but you just can't get anywhere?

About 4 months into my new dream job at Discovery, it was clear that while I loved the company and the people, my opportunity for my creative dream to flourish was not in alignment. It was like I was in the right Church but the wrong pew. I was mystified.

I mean "Lord Universe...!! I did the work...I took the fear leap into the great abandon...and then.... nada? That was not in the rule book."

As the time wore on, I got more frustrated. I wanted to trust the universe, but the doubt slowly began to take over. Time went on. By day, I worked on one meaningless project after another. By night, I decided to use my time alone in my apartment to map out my big idea. Surely that would be the key. Take ACTION. Do the research. Figure out the shows. Get the pitch deck ready. SEE IT.

The summer came and it was time for my family to join me in Maryland, where we were looking for a home close to the Discovery Headquarters in Silver Spring. The Dallas house sold. Our furniture was shipped to a Maryland storage facility and my husband and son were ready to head to Silver Spring to start house hunting. That's when Ralph got word from his HR office that they would not let his job transfer to Maryland. "Excuse me?" I said, trying to decipher the impact of this new information on our plans. "Our furniture has already been shipped here...how can they just change their minds like that. "I don't know," Ralph said. "They've given me two options. To either stay in Texas or go back to the NJ office."

Well, there's a miscalculation. My job was nowhere near those two places. What now, oh great and powerful universe?

As I stood in the shower trying to think through our options, I asked my spirit team for guidance. As the warm water cascaded over my ears, I heard the words (as god is my witness, I literally heard them) "You have to go to New York."

Eureka! Well of course, I thought. That all makes sense! That's why I didn't feel right. I'm in the right church, it's just that my pew is in NYC. Of course!

With renewed optimism, I went to my boss at Discovery and explained the situation. "Work from the NYC office, Karen. We need someone there anyway. In fact, it'll help the team to have you there."

Well now you're talking Universe! Pivot, bank, shoot, score!!

In the end, the solution was better than perfect. We moved back to the same NJ town that we had lived in before moving to Texas, as we felt this was the best for Graham, who was starting high school. He was more than excited to get back to his childhood stomping ground and be back with his grade school friends. Ralph had a twenty-minute drive to his AT&T office where he reunited with old friends and colleagues. All seemed right with the world again.

And my pitch deck was done. And it was good. It visualized taking one of Discovery's smaller channels and re-imagining it as a lifestyle channel. In essence, taking many of the Oprah inspired spiritual ideas, and marrying them with the explorative curiosity of the science channel. To further integrate the Discovery brand genres, I also sprinkled in some mediums, ghost exploration, wholistic eating and feng shui. I had designed the network of television that I wanted to watch... and I knew I could sell it.

I was ready for my moment.

And that's when I got my chance.

Understanding the Formula of Manifestation

So, here's the thing. Having a passion is great. Having a vision of what you want to create is also great. But I want to stand here and tell you that it is really important to consider one of the biggest lessons that Wayne Dyer taught me. No matter what, you have to have a mind that is open to everything and attached to nothing.

Why? Because sometimes the universe has an even better idea than you do. It is the Universe after all. And you need to allow it to do its thing.

It bears repeating:

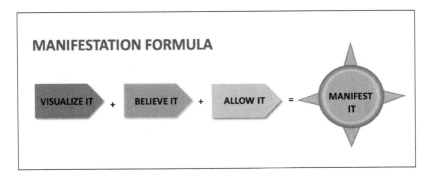

I'll explain how.

I don't know about you, but the power of the thoughts in my head downright scares me. Sometimes it really feels like I'm just a bystander in someone else's head.... it's true that we are all our worst self-critics and yet, why do we continue those repetitive thoughts of self-blame, doubt and criticism about ourselves?

I have found that the most effective way for eliminating the fear and self-doubt talk in my head and to activate the positives of my purpose is through affirmations.

Just – Say – What – I – Want (so there is no confusion, right universe?).

Some would say, affirm what you do want, and cancel out what you don't.

I learned this from the best. No one understood the power of affirmations better than Louise Hay.

The Mother of Affirmations:

It was the summer of 1988 and I was living in St Louis, when I got a frantic call from my sister. "Mom's really lost it this time," Diane said. "And this is new?" I asked.

My mother, as I have shared with you, was always into doing things that were 'out there.'

Diane, who was still living at home at the time, wasn't having it. "She just packed her bags and left for California." "What??" I asked, suddenly feeling my sarcasm leap to confusion. "Yes, she's gone to some self-healing affirmation seminar that's run by a new age crazy woman who makes people speak into mirrors and say they love themselves. I mean who does that?" "Mom does," I said, silently intrigued.

That was the beginning of what I like to call my mother's foray into Louis Hay. And while those were the very early days, as many of you already know, Louise would later become the crowned majesty of the new age movement. She had just published the New York Times best seller, "You Can Heal Your Life" which would ultimately launch the multi-million dollar, global publishing business, Hay House.

Louise had an incredible story. She had an incredibly difficult early life that was scarred by an abusive father, and being sexually assaulted when she was sixteen. She dropped out of school and gave birth to a daughter, her only child, whom she gave up for adoption. Louise later moved to NYC and became a fashion model. She married, and then divorced fourteen years later, when her husband left her for another woman.

Lost and alone, Louise volunteered to work at the Science of Mind Church in Manhattan, where she began to learn and understand the power of the mind. She learned transcendental meditation. And then, another life milestone, a cancer diagnosis, required Louise to apply those same tools and principles to aid in her own self-healing. Six months later, Louise was pronounced "cancer free" by her doctors. Louise compiled these insights into a book about how our thoughts and beliefs can manifest as a physical effect on the body as "dis-ease."

That book would become the international sensation, "You Can Heal Your Life." "Now I knew from personal experience," Louise would write "That dis-ease can be healed if we are willing to change the way we think and believe and act." Louise soon began helping others use positive affirmations to overcome and improve their lives.

Here are some of Louise's points of philosophy directly from the first chapter of that book. See if any of these ring true for you.

1. The Point of Power is always in the present moment
2. Every thought we think is creating our future
3. The only thing we are ever dealing with is a thought and a thought can be changed
4. We can change our attitude about the past
5. To release the past, we must be willing to forgive
6. We must be willing to begin to learn to love ourselves.

Louise's work would inspire millions of followers and new writers and teachers as the seeds of their own spiritual growth and transformation.

How Affirmations Work

Very soon after my mom came back from her Louise Hay getaway, our house was covered with affirmations like the following:

> I am willing to change
> I am willing to ask for help when I need it.
> I release all drama from my life
> There is always more to learn
> I express love and gratitude for the blessings in my life

"I am willing to release affirmations created by my mother which are attempting to control my behavior."

An affirmation, according to Louise, is really *anything you say or think*. By definition, an affirmation is a declaration that something exists, or is true. And science tells us that we think over 50,000 thoughts per day. Think about the power of that! Those declarations, if said often enough, become our beliefs.

Whether we realize it or not, most of us are constantly stating affirmations in our minds every day. Unfortunately, a lot of what we normally think and say to ourselves can be quite negative, which is not going to bring us the positive experiences we want. Retraining ourselves to catch that thinking and speaking positive thoughts in our minds is the key to manifesting the wonderful lives and futures that we want.

Mind-Wrestling with Your Subconscious

According to Louise, "an affirmation opens the door to your subconscious mind by consciously choosing to think positive thoughts. It's a beginning point on the path to change. 'When I talk about *doing affirmations,' Louise wrote,* 'I mean consciously choosing words that will either help *eliminate* something from your life or help *create* something new in your life.'

Some people say that "affirmations don't work" (which is an affirmation in itself), when what they mean is that they don't know how to use them correctly. They may say, *"My prosperity is growing,"* but then think, *Oh, this is stupid, I know it won't work.* Which affirmation do you think will win out? The negative one, of course, because it's part of a long-standing, habitual way of looking at life. Sometimes people will say their affirmations once a day and complain the rest of the time. It will take a long time for affirmations to work if they're done that way. The complaining affirmations will always win, because there are more of them and they're usually said with great feeling.'"

Louise believed that if we could eliminate negative self-talk and replace it with a positive statement that it had transformational power. Sounds simple, but oh so hard to keep our thoughts positive when life hands out those lemons. But if "thoughts are things" and "what we think is what we get" are the magic building blocks for creating the life we want, then the tools for distilling and shifting that self-talk to achieve our new direction and outcome, must be placed and activated within our Lifemap. This is the place where you lock your GPS to your true north star.

My goal is to help you spotlight the spaces that you've identified that have already influenced you by maximizing the positive and cancelling out the negative. So you will look to the sun and turn your back on the shadow. Because, and you already know this... what you focus on grows.

So, let's cull your garden.

LIFEMAPPING EXPLORATION #9:

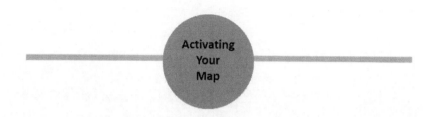

This is where the magic happens...where your map reveals its story...this is where we take the incredible work that you did in the last chapter of laying out your lifemap and here we simplify the story to show you what you came to learn and what you came to do.

This next step in your revelation exercise will help you to cull the key elements from your Lifemapping Landscape and find the most important clues for what you are here to know and learn.

There are many different feelings and beliefs that have no doubt surfaced for you within each category, that are all relevant whispers about your souls' purpose. As you read through what you've written as your lessons of Love and Fear from your Life Milestones, Lessons from your Soul Squad and your insights from What You Love To Do, you'll start to see reoccurring themes that are threaded through your "I am" statements.

The key themes are:

1. What you came to **Teach, Be and Give** = LOVE
2. What you came to **Learn, Overcome and Release** = FEAR

As you review, you'll find that you have probably written similar forms of the same feelings and beliefs in your FEAR columns, such as:

"I am a coward. I'm not smart. I am unloved."

This is what you have come to learn, overcome and release. Similarly, you'll may also find similar themes, ideas or feelings pop up in your LOVE columns...

"I am a seeker." "I am an explorer." "I am a learner."

This is a theme around what you have come to be, teach and give. The idea of this exercise is to simplify your story. To select 3 Key "I am" statements that you feel ring truest for you and bounce up the strongest vibrations on your love and fear scale. These are the beckoning's of your life's purpose.

Calling in Your Angels of Inspiration

To ground before you begin, consider this Soulfirmation that specifically calls upon your angels and guides to assist you in seeing those key insights and life lessons that are most important for you to know, action and understand right now.

For a moment, close your eyes, and visualize your spirit team around you, happy that you have called them in to help you with this important exercise. They know and understand your pure, divine higher self, and what it is that you most want to learn and offer the world.

Listen with your heart for their guidance, and as they help channel and energize your inner knowingness for the truth to speak to you.

Take a deep breath in...holding it a moment as you feel their strength around you.... and then, release, slowly and deeply, releasing into the knowingness that you are surrounded with love.

 SOULFIRMATION #10

"Underneath,
All of the things that life has taught me about myself
I remember who I am.
I am there steeped in the murmurings of my heart
Waiting to be heard.
In the stillness of the asking, I can hear the whisper of my soul
Affirming everything I've ever known...everything I've ever been...everything I am.
I am Whole.
I am aligned. I am balanced. I am certain.
I shine brightly in my own light
Just as I am...Just as I have always been.
Affirming and aligning with those who are always with me.
I am only a stranger to the world...
I am a seeker looking out of my own eyes.
And I see me.
I see exactly who I am.
I am perfect. I am eternal. I am love ."

Tallying Your Key Takeaways:

Here you'll take the expanded view of your lifemap and break it down to the 3 key insights *from each Love/Fear experience that stands out as the key life lessons for you.*

Here are the steps to get there.

- **Step #1: Review**: Go back to your fully expanded view of your Lifemap on page ## in Chapter 9. Carefully read through all of the I am statements.

- **Step #2: Reflect:** Spend some time asking your soul guides to help you identify the underlying themes that reoccur most often in your map.

- **Step #3: Choose:** Circle or highlight the statements that stand out the most. A clue is that the themes the reoccur the most are probably the ones that need the most attention. Narrow down your selections into your "3 Key Takeaways."

- **Step #4: Transfer:** Take your top 3 I am statements and place them on the chart on pg. ## know that you can adapt and adjust your I am statements however you feel they best fit into these categories. **You can re-write** them if you want to adjust your statements differently within this context, or if you need to restate them to combine ideas into a single phrase.

For help, I have also added a copy of my own Lifemapping exercise for your reference on page 286.

When you complete this exercise, we'll be creating these statements into activating affirmations for you to chart your life map forward.

Alrighty - Here is your Lifemapping Reminder for this exploration.

Lifemapping Reminder:

1. **20 minutes** is a good time limit for this exploration
2. In this exercise, if you can **light a candle** for this intention, it will remind you of the light within you.
3. **Keep your journal close** in case any insights, feelings or thoughts come to you from your inner self or your soul guides that you may want to capture.
4. Continue to **breathe deeply** as you go. Inhaling energy and exhaling anything you want to release as you contemplate these significant life moments from your soul journey.

Now, off you go!

MY LIFE MAP: Key Takeaways

Key in on the top 3 takeaways from your Lifemapping exercise.

THINGS I LEARNED FROM MY LOVE MILESTONES	THINGS I LEARNED FROM MY FEAR MILESTONES	THINGS I LEARNED FROM MY LOVE SQUAD	THINGS I LEARNED FROM MY FEAR SQUAD	THINGS I'M GOOD AT (DO WITH LOVE)	THINGS THAT CHALLENGE or PREVENT ME FROM DOING WHAT I LOVE
1.	1.	1.	1.	1.	1.
2.	2.	2.	2.	2.	2.
3.	3.	3.	3.	3.	3.
What I Need to Teach	What I Need to Learn	Who I Came to Be	What I Came to Overcome	What I Need to Give	What I Need to Release

And for reference, here's mine to share.

MY LIFE MAP: Key Takeaways

Key in on the top 3 takeaways from your Lifemapping exercise.

THINGS I LEARNED FROM MY LOVE MILESTONES	THINGS I LEARNED FROM MY FEAR MILESTONES	THINGS I LEARNED FROM MY LOVE SQUAD	THINGS I LEARNED FROM MY FEAR SQUAD	THINGS I'M GOOD AT (DO WITH LOVE)	THINGS THAT CHALLENGE or PREVENT ME FROM DOING WHAT I LOVE
1. I am strong	1. I am a harsh judge of myself	1. I am a storyteller	1. I am not smart enough	1. I am a talented writer/producer	1. I could fail
2. I am intuitive	2. I am afraid to fail	2. I am a teacher	2. I am not talented enough	2. I love learning and sharing spiritual concepts and ideas	2. I might not have enough talent
3. I am an uplifter	3. I am afraid of being judged by others	3. I am a seeker	3. I am not brave enough	3. I'm a good at inspiring people and elevating their energy	3. I might be too old
What I Need to Teach	What I Need to Learn	Who I Came to Be	What I Came to Overcome	What I Need to Give	What I Need to Release

Holy moly love, you are amazing!! This is like getting a soul makeover.

This is you at your essence.... the "essential" you! And you look marvelous!

My guess is that you may have gone in and rewritten some of your "I am" statements in this section to really capture the essence of your top 3 statements, and that is exactly the right way to think about this exercise.

It's also important to really stop and think about these statements and what feelings, memories, and ideas they evoke within you. Can you imagine the conversation that you may have had with your angels and guides before stepping into this lifetime, and what experiences and lessons you wanted to learn?

Does this help you see a better vision of why you are here?

Later in this chapter, you are going to work these statements all into affirmations of love and use them as the tools that will help you to map out your future?

I can't wait to see where you will go next!

A Seeker's Story:

As you get closer to clarifying and identifying the life-learnings from your map, you will find that you recognize and know more than ever before what you have come to Teach, Learn and Be, as well as what you need to Overcome, Give and Release.

This inner clarity may start as a tiny yearning that grows into full-fledged calling. And when the calling beckons in its proud, clear voice, it's time to brush away fear and run towards the truth. This is what happened to my friend Jena Coray, when she let her passion rule and lead her towards her true purpose of helping others heal and find their own voices within.

As you read through Jena's story...look for the clues she followed in her own milestones that lead her to her to discovering her life's purpose.

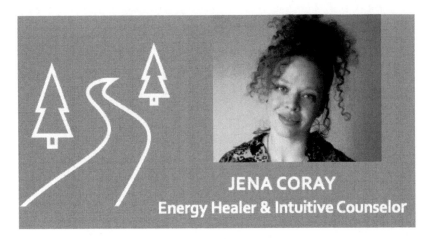

JENA CORAY
Energy Healer & Intuitive Counselor

I felt the nervousness in my gut, first. Then, shaky knees as I walked up to my boss' desk. I had spent nearly three years in that cubicle, when the plan was for it to be a summer job stint between degrees. I didn't know I'd meet the love of my life there and decide to stay for a while. Or that from the mind-numbing tedium that the job entailed, I'd be pressurized into becoming the shining diamond of myself.

From the confines of that cube, my creativity burst into a passion project, turned side-hustle, turned full-fledged moonlighting situation. The perceived security of my day job had begun to feel like chains holding me back from what I was really meant to be, do and have. I was ready to break free. To trust myself. To love myself enough to chase my dreams and follow my deep, soul yearnings.

"I am ready to do this. I am here to help others. I am ready to be the healer and teacher that I know I've come here to be."

I spoke from an anxious, racing heart as I told my boss I was ready to commit to my vision full time and was giving my two weeks notice.

Immediately, I felt a wave of freedom and relief rushing through my body. I have faithfully pursued my dreams from that day forward and it has opened me up to a more beautiful, purposeful, magical life than I ever knew was possible.

Today's Jena's Energy practice Mo MOJO.com is thriving. She's helping thousands of her clients around the world shift their energy and teach them how to shed the false beliefs that are holding them back and find the magic within themselves.

And I'm not gonna throw away my shot...

It was that kind of "go for it" determination that locked my throttle into high gear as I walked into the office of Karen Leever. Karen had just joined Discovery as an Executive Vice President and was brand new to the NYC office when I nervously tapped on her door. I had been following the news that she had been chosen to come in and revamp the struggling digital side of the business. She had a big job in front of her.

After I had gotten the go ahead to move from the Silver Spring, Maryland office to New York, I had rewired my mental mindset. My family had happily relocated back to NJ and began braving the two-and-a-half-hour commute into the city. I was getting up at 4:45 a.m. which gave me enough time for a sprint on the treadmill, a fast spritz in the shower and make a mad dash to the station to catch the six o'clock train to Manhattan. If all went well, I got to my desk by 8:30 a.m. It was a stressful, arduous, and exhausting journey, but I was determined that this was my time. If I had the courage to just "go for it," I knew that the road would become clear.

Anyone who knows me would vouch for the fact that the brazen courage it took for me to walk into Karen's office was not in my typical nature. But I remember hearing/feeling/ knowing that this was my shot…. and nothing was going to stop me from throwing it as far and as hard as I could.

I was fortunate to arrive that morning when I did. It was before 9:00 a.m. and the entire office floor was virtually empty. Karen warmly offered the chair in front of her desk to me, as I introduced myself. For twenty minutes, I shared the story of why I came to Discover… my vision, my passion for telling stories and creating content so closely aligned with the Discovery brands, that I was certain could reach a whole new audience in a whole new way. She carefully reviewed my pitch deck and my idea of how we could leverage both the linear TV and new streaming platforms and dig into the treasure trove of the Discovery library to create both long and short form shows.

I showed her the data I had pulled together around the exploding growth of mindfulness content. How more and more young people were turning to older "traditions and practices," because they were seeking meaning and purpose. Practices like meditation, yoga and wholistic eating and products were booming. People are looking for meaning today more than ever," I told her. How is it that Discovery's umbrella brand, with channels like Science Channel, Food Network, Travel Channel, and HGTV, is not the one to take the lead in showing young people where astrology comes from, how to make organic food, or how to design your home around fengshui. No one is doing that, and audiences are hungry for this kind of real-life television." I said.

Karen got it. "I love it," she said. "But I'm really new here, and have been given a very specific job to do. Perhaps we can give this some focus after I get the core Discovery digital channels launched successfully?"

"Oh my gosh," I thought to myself as I shook Karen's hand, thanking her for her time. She heard me!

As I walked out to the elevator, my heart thumped in my chest like a had just ran another marathon. My head spun as I replayed our conversation, laughing out loud at the brazen audacity I had to take that walk and sell my idea. But did it ever feel GOOD to look fear in the face and do it anyway. It was another finish line that would open up another test of my endurance.

No one ever said that being brave was the same as being fearless.

The great news is Karen gave me the job as her head of Digital Operations and over time, we forged a kind of ying/ yang relationship where she brought her strong, fiercely intellectual and strategic thinking, and I brought the uplift- ing, encouraging, cheerleading, inspired-belief. It turned out that we rode the same train line to work every day, so we would meet up over coffee at the station in the morning, that would take us to Penn Station, then to the E train 5 stops to 3rd Avenue to our office in mid-town. In the intensity of the pressure and brain numbing stress, we developed a deep friendship, like two battle buddies on the front line.

While Karen did an amazing job building out the business, I tried to learn everything I could about creating and deliv- ering digital content. Slowly, my Mind Body Spirit Channel was evolving into a digital platform. On the long train rides home from work, I reformatted and reworked the vision over and over in my mind. I imagined how far reaching and impactful it could be if this could be a personalized experience. With access to shows, books, classes, movies, even live communities of people iterating, learning, connecting and finding like-minded connections all around the world.

To my delight, I had gotten to part 2 of the manifestation process.

I could SEE IT/VISUALIZE IT + BELIEVE IT

I was 100% there. With every ounce of my being. I was riding high on the manifestation train, waiting for the mighty Universe to deliver.

It was all I could do to stay patient.... the vision was so real. But the universe remained silent. In the meantime, I worked on every other kind of project...looking for the crack of light that I was certain would seed the womb of my Discovery/Oprah conception. But all the doors remained shut. Weeks and months stretched on into a truly dark night of the soul.

Once again, I inwardly yelled at the unyielding Universe. I could not understand why this huge vision had been placed in my heart...that I could SEE it so clearly in my mind. Why wasn't I creating it? It was like it was a locked door waiting for a key to be found. It was an ache I felt in my chest, and I was getting tired.

It was around that time that the movie *La La Land* came out. By myself in a darkened theatre, I watched the story unfold about a young musician and actress trying and failing to find success in Hollywood. Towards the end of the movie, the leading lady, Mia, who has given everything to get her break and is ready to give up, makes one last audition for a movie that was going to be filmed in Paris. When asked to tell a personal story about herself, Mia shares that she'd had an aunt who once lived in Paris, and sings a song called "Here's to the Ones who Dream."

As I listened to the lyrics feeling the words searing through my heart, I began to quietly sob alone in the darkness, feeling the loss of my own dying dream. Of the years of work, moving my family across the country...hardly ever seeing them with my long hours away, commuting back and forth on the train. My son growing up without me being home for dinner. My husband bearing the burden of fulfilling the role of both mother and father. Of the endless hours, dedication, effort, stress, and getting nowhere. "Here's to the ones who dream..." Mia sang through in her audition. "Foolish as they may seem...here's to the ones that ache. Here's to the mess we make." The lyrics of that song were like a knife through my fledgling spirit. Like a last crashing wave fighting to land on the sand only to fall short and ebb back into the sea.

"Why was I cursed with this stupid dream?" I wondered. "Why couldn't I just give up, and forget it?" I felt like a lost explorer, floating without direction to a destination that I KNEW was out there, drifting further and further away from my discovery in darkness.

I drove from the movie that night, feeling like Mia, like was time to let it all go. It felt like a dull, tired ache...that needed to be snuffed out, so I could let go of the pain of it.

Little did I know that was on the verge of the final magical ingredient I needed to activate my manifestation.

SEE IT/VISUALIZE IT + BELIEVE IT + ALLOW IT = MANIFEST IT

"Allowing" meant, I had to let it go.

What was the old saying? "If you love something, set it free. If it comes back to you, it's yours. If it doesn't, it never was." That was from the incredible book, Jonathan Livingston Seagull, a classic story, about a bird with a dream who would not settle for an ordinary life. Thank you, Richard Bach.

Little did I know that the Universe was helping me to reshape my life map in a whole new way...and was about to give me an opportunity to reaffirm who I was, that would reshape all my beliefs, lives and fears in ways I never could have dreamed of.

Like Jonathan Livingston Seagull, it was time for me to fly.

 SOUL GOODY BAG

Here are some resources mentioned in this chapter for you for further exploration:

- **You Can Heal Your Life by Louise Hay** - Louise Hay, bestselling author, is an internationally known leader in the self-help field. Her key message is: "If we are willing to do the mental work, almost anything can be healed. Through Louise's healing techniques and positive philosophy, millions have learned how to create more of what they want in their lives, including more wellness in their bodies, minds, and spirits.

- **The Power is Within You by Louise Hay** - In this book, Louise Hay expands her philosophies of loving the self through learning to listen and trust the inner voice, loving the child within, letting our true feelings out, expressing our creativity, creating a world that is ecologically sound where it's safe to love each other and much more.

- **Jonathan Livingston Seagull by Richard Bach -** This is a story for people who follow their hearts and make their own rules...people who get special pleasure out of doing something well, even if only for themselves... people who know there's more to this *living* than meets the eye: they'll be right there with Jonathan, flying higher and faster than ever they dreamed.

- **Jena Coray** – Jena life's work is dedicated to help people who are ready to create more balance, ease and freedom in their lives, from the inside out. Through energetic healing and intuitive practice, dedicated self-care and emotional awareness, and by busting through old patterns & mental blocks, she completely changed her own life and her ability to flow through all the ups and downs life brings with more ease, clarity & acceptance. Now she's dedicated to integrating these energetic, intuitive & mindset shifting practices into everyday life and be a guide to help light to help those seeking their true selves to BE all who've come to Earth to be. Find Jena here getmomojo.com.

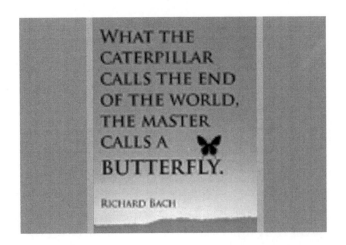

WHAT THE CATERPILLAR CALLS THE END OF THE WORLD, THE MASTER CALLS A BUTTERFLY.

RICHARD BACH

CHAPTER 11

DEFINING YOUR PATH FORWARD

Two years to the day after taking on my new job at Discovery, my boss called me into her office. With a serious look, she asked me to sit in that same chair in front of her desk where we had our first conversation together.

"I just got a phone call," she said with suddenly mischievously look in her eyes. "Turns out Ms. Winfrey wants a plan for building a digital platform."

At first, I couldn't understand what she was talking about. "The Oprah Winfrey Network already has its own digital app where you can watch her TV shows," I responded.

"Apparently, she wants to create a different kind of experience," Karen continued. "That takes her Super Soul Sunday programming, the Oprah Show and Oprah Magazine content and brings it all together into one experience." Karen paused for a moment, allowing the weight of her statement to sink in, and then looked at me straight in the eye. "Sound like some kind of mind, body, spirit platform. I wonder who on my team would want to work on something like that?"

Holy mother boatload of affirmations! Wait, I thought I had given up?

I hadn't given up- I had just let go. I went from mandate to manifest, all by simply allowing it into being. And it landed like a butterfly on my shoulder.

My Manifestation Motherload

Two weeks later, I was seated in Oprah Winfrey's conference room at OWN: The Oprah Winfrey Network's headquarters in Los Angeles. Sitting at the table was the OWN counsel of content elders. The President of OWN, the Executive Producer of *Super Soul Sunday,* the editor and chief of *O, The Oprah Magazine* and more senior executives. We were all gathered for a communal brainstorm about the idea of launching the first app of its kind with Discovery.

During that meeting, I was seated directly across from a stunning woman who introduced herself as Robyn Miller Brecker. At first glance, I thought she might be talent from one of OWN's new shows. She had such a sparkling aura to her, a warm, reassuring friendliness that made me feel welcome and "seen." She was clearly part of the pack that had gathered for this meeting, and her quick smile put me at ease in that powerful room.

Robyn had been on Oprah's team for over 20 years and had launched her entire digital platform, oprah.com, including all the online events and workshops that had introduced me to some of my biggest "aha moments," including the New Earth online webcast with Eckart Tolle. Robyn and I would become digital partners on the OWN app project, but little did we know that universe had a much higher purpose for the both of us in mind.

Winks from the Universe

Four months later, I was back in LA. It was the evening before the big in-person pitch meeting with Oprah. I remember looking out the window at the Hollywood Hills, really understanding for the first time what so many dreamers felt like before the big audition. It was a city built on wishes and work. Passions and prayer. The city of angels indeed.

As I settled in, I asked for those angels to come and help me be a good steward of the right words that would make Oprah fall in love with our idea. I felt so good about what we'd put together. I had rehearsed every word. I was ready... It was like the night before giving birth to a brand-new baby...my Oprah Discovery baby. My heart was ready to burst with gratitude.

I grabbed my journal to capture my feelings on paper, so I'd always be able to replay the moment. I opened it up on a page I'd written two year's prior. "Today I met Wayne Dwyer in person at the Louise Hay, You Can Do It Conference, in Austin Texas!" Of all things to read I thought...

That event had become another life-changing milestone in my life. It was two months after the Boston Marathon, and I was still riding high on the adrenaline of my new outlook, when I accepted a last-minute invite from my friend Kim to attend the event with her. The keynote speaker was Wayne Dyer, and I had never heard him speak in person.

Kim was my feisty Texan friend, who at the time, was working for Mark Cuban at ASX TV in Dallas. We both splurged on upgraded tickets and hung on Wayne's every word. I smiled, re-reading some of the quotes that I captured from him in that journal.

"We have been raised to believe in our ordinary-ness. In order to get past ordinary, you have to let go of the things that you believe are true."

Thanks Wayne. I felt like every word was just for me.

Used to celebrity wrangling, Kim was able to convince the event manager to let me go backstage and meet Wayne in person. In a moment that felt like a miracle, I was able to tell him the influence that his writings and meditations had in my life, that inspired me with the vision of creating a global television network for bringing inspirational, mindful, spiritual, conscious, life expanding and enlightening programming to people around the world.

"My dear," Wayne said, like a father speaking to a daughter. "If you see it, you will create it. It's the law of the universe."

Reading those words again, the night before meeting Oprah, where I was going to unveil such a vision, took my breath away. "Thanks for sending me that sign, Wayne." I smiled. And then I almost dropped the book. The date of the entry was June 11, 2015. The next day's date with Oprah? June 11, 2018!!

Three years to the day, I had fulfilled my affirmation of actually doing this. Tears of gratitude streamed from my eyes. It felt as if Wayne was in the room with me, letting me know that he was rooting for me. Everything had **finally** aligned.

I was about to see my dream come true.

Back to Your Future

As we continue to build and simplify our life map vision utilizing the very important foundation of our past love and fear that have been part of our journey and belief system, we will continue to break them down into one simplified vision, using tools that you can practice every day to speak your vision into being. And we will do it consciously so that it gives you both power and peace.

In this chapter we will:

- **Activate and Re-Calibrate Your Intentions:** Now that you've prioritized your top "I am" statements, we will supercharge them into powerful and purposeful affirmations that will help energize and uplift you to put you in the "positive receiving mode" of your dreams.

    This is the place where you will harness the power of "I am" by

    - Developing an affirmation mindset that will help you keep your positive thoughts and energy in check and to cancel out the negativity.
    - Choosing and affirming what you want, and letting go of what you don't.
    - Understanding how to use fear, doubt and uncertainty as your power.
    - Learning how to re-Invent and re-envision the future you want when things don't go as planned.

- **Create your Own Personalized Soul-firmation:** This is your unique statement of purpose that reflects all of your experiences, lessons and beliefs in one place. You can affirm, tweak, edit and affirm this as your life's purpose evolves and emerges.

- **Articulate Your Story:** Once you are in the powerful receiving mode of the I am energy, we'll take one last leap together on to the stage of the spoken word, where you will use your voice to send your dreams out into the universe, into the manifestation zone.

Activate and Calibrate to Create Your Dreams

So, we're going to do three super powerful things.

1. First, we are going to **ACTIVATE** (ignite/Increase/ amplify its power) everything about what you are here **to teach, to be and to do more of.**
2. Second, we are going to **RECALLIBRATE** (readjust/ decrease/diminish its power) the things that you are *learning, working on and releasing.*
3. And third, we are going to **CREATE** powerful, positive statements that you can use every day, that will **activate and calibrate your intentions at a soul level** to shine the light on that seedling of your vision within your soul, so you can prune, grow and water whatever serves you best now into your wonderful, fulfilling future.

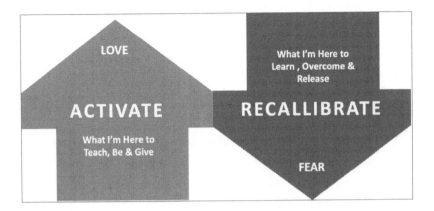

As you begin to really identify and align with the things that you know are your connections with the feelings and actions that affirm the feeling of LOVE, these are where we will shine a light, so that they become a loving focal point of your daily intentions. Likewise, as you identify those things that have taught you fear-based beliefs or feelings that you do NOT want, we will work on restating or recalibrating the energy around those beliefs, to disengage their negative power over you, and realign them with the "I am" power of love.

And again, for the most part, this is a simple transfer of the work you've already done. Ready? This is the home stretch!!

LIFEMAPPING EXPLORATION #10 – Part 1

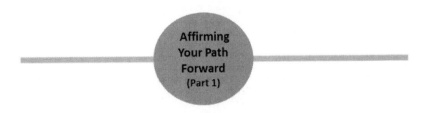

Here's the plan:

- **Step #1** –Fill in your Top 3 Love and Fear Key Takeaways in your love and fear categories into the page below.

- **Step #2** - Then take each thought in your Love sections and make it a positive statement. For example: "I am a good visualizer" becomes "I am a visionary." As much as possible, use "I am" to affirm the things you love about yourself and the things that really capture the heart of who you are. When this section is complete, it should reflect the qualities about you that make you feel good/empowered/en-lightened.

- **Step #3** – Do the same with your Fear section. In this case, rather than making it an "I am" statement, take your Fear thought and flip it into a positive statement. For example: Instead of "I tend to be overly self-critical" flip it to the positive: "I love myself fully."

Continue to work through this exercise until you have a full view of how you are going to activate the love affirmations and recalibrate the fear affirmations into new beacons of light energy. Read those bottom 9 affirmations carefully... these are what you have come to learn, be and practice. And if you can get to a place where those affirmations become your reality, ah, what an amazing life review it will be!

I've placed my Lifemap Purpose Affirmations Exercise for you to review on page 305 as an example. This is what it will look like when you are done. You're taking your "Key Takeaways" and creating your affirmation statements.

Your Lifemapping Reminder is the same as our prior exercises only in this case, you will be creating your own Soul-firmation at the end that takes all of your "I am" statements into one wholistic story. Your picture is now coming to life.

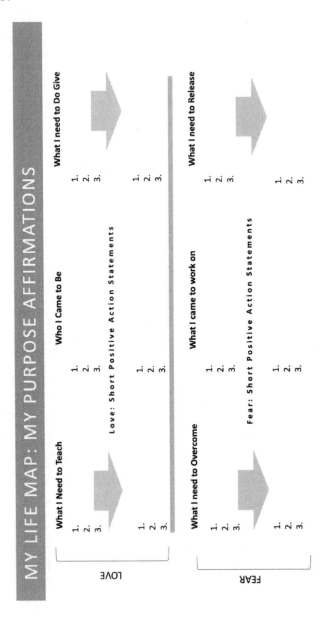

Here is my Lifemap Purpose Exploration that you can reference as an example.

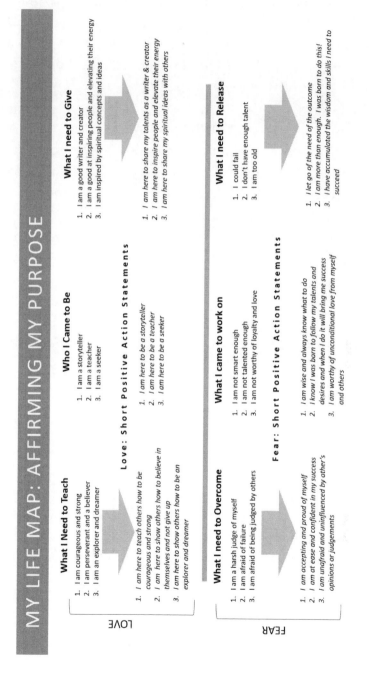

MY LIFE MAP: AFFIRMING MY PURPOSE

What I Need to Teach
1. I am courageous and strong
2. I am perseverant and a believer
3. I am an explorer and dreamer

Who I Came to Be
1. I am a storyteller
2. I am a teacher
3. I am a seeker

What I need to Give
1. I am a good writer and creator
2. I am a good at inspiring people and elevating their energy
3. I am inspired by spiritual concepts and ideas

Love: Short Positive Action Statements

1. I am here to teach others how to be courageous and strong
2. I am here to show others how to believe in themselves and not give up
3. I am here to show others how to be an explorer and dreamer

1. I am here to be a storyteller
2. I am here to be a teacher
3. I am here to be a seeker

1. I am here to share my talents as a writer & creator
2. I am here to inspire people and elevate their energy
3. I am here to share my spiritual ideas with others

What I need to Overcome
1. I am a harsh judge of myself
2. I am afraid of failure
3. I am afraid of being judged by others

What I came to work on
1. I am not smart enough
2. I am not talented enough
3. I am not worthy of loyalty and love

What I need to Release
1. I could fail
2. I don't have enough talent
3. I am too old

Fear: Short Positive Action Statements

1. I am accepting and proud of myself
2. I am at ease and confident in my success
3. I am unafraid and uninfluenced by other's opinions or judgements

1. I am wise and always know what to do
2. I know I was born to follow my talents and desires and when I do it will bring me success
3. I am worthy of unconditional love from myself and others

1. I let go of the need of the outcome
2. I am more than enough. I was born to do this!
3. I have accumulated the wisdom and skills I need to succeed

LOVE

FEAR

Meeting Oprah

I don't remember sleeping but I awoke to the perfect California day just in time to watch the sun rise. My mother called to wish me luck and walked me through an affirmation mediation with Marianne Williamson, that quieted my nerves and boosted my confidence.

I was ready.

I can honestly say that during our meeting there was never a moment of doubt in my mind. Robyn gave me a wink of confidence as Oprah sat down, looking just as I expected...perfectly put together. Upbeat, expectant, in business mode. Ready to hear the pitch.

My boss, Karen, began the presentation, reviewing the strategy, the numbers and the target audience. And then it was my turn.

I can't tell you what a thrill it is to be able to say thank you to your hero for bringing them every book, author and idea that helped not only me, but a whole generation of seekers. And what a privilege it was to be able to present her with a tool that I believed could inspire and introduce new young seekers to content that they many never have discovered, unless Discovery and Oprah came together to present it in a whole new way.

This idea would help open up the world by giving them unlimited access to content personalized just for them... in the way they wanted to consume it or discover it. "So many of your ideas were ahead of their time," I said to Ms. Winfrey, meaning every word. "And now the world needs this more than ever."

We played a little video segment showing Oprah the magic of how we could re-edit some of her most powerful and profound teachings and ideas. One clip featured her answering one of my very favorite questions. It was hard for me not to choke up listening to her watching it play on the conference room screen. For me, it summed up how I had gotten to that room in the first place. It was in Oprah's own voice summing up the equation for manifestation.

"How do you find the balance between making things happen and letting things happen? "You do all that you can do. You do the work. You prepare. You get Ready for the opportunity to step in. And then you let it go. You release all attachment to the outcome."

VISUALIZE IT + BELIEVE IT + ALLOW IT = MANIFEST IT

The feedback on the meeting was really good. Karen and I celebrated with a glass of wine at the beautiful Shutters Hotel in Santa Monica before grabbing our flight back to New York. We waited for the green light.

Four days later, Apple announced a multi-year streaming deal with Oprah Winfrey. My heart sank upon hearing of this collaboration.... our mind, body, spirit app was dead.

I felt like my soul had been ripped out of my chest. I simply couldn't believe it. This couldn't possibly be IT??!! No way, not after all of the work ...all the *following my heart* and *listening to my inner voice*... they led me all the way across the country! I had put my whole self out there ...I had sat across the table from Oprah herself and boldly pitched an idea that had taken me *years* to birth. After holding my newborn baby in my arms just 4 days prior, I had just been given word that it was dead. I felt as if the rug had been pulled out from underneath me. I felt sick and deceived ...like the universe was playing a cruel trick on me.

Any yet, there it was.

Every ounce of my newfound faith in the universe crashed. Hard. The "no," singeing the very fabric of my soul.

When God shuts a door, he always opens up a window

I got on a conference call early the next week with Robyn to do an adeptly named "postmortem" call, which meant officially taking the family of product designers and developers off the project. Everyone was disappointed. Many had discovered Orpah's content for the first time and had become true believers that we were working on something that would have a meaningful impact.

The only one that was upbeat on the call was Robyn. She was talking about her upcoming article on Oprah.com called "The Night A Medium Changed My Life." The team was immediately fascinated. "Don't worry," Robyn said. "I'll be talking more about it on my show."

"What show?"

I called Robyn back after the conference call ended. "What did you mean when you said, 'I'll be talking more about it on your show?'"

Robyn laughed. "I can't believe that I actually said that out loud." Robyn went on to tell me that it was her intention to leave OWN and start her own company. "The article will explain everything." She spoke. "I'll send it to you."

The article told the story of how Robyn's dad had passed very suddenly when she was 12, leaving a huge void in her family's life. It wasn't until years later that she was able to reconnect with him through a spiritual medium, and it changed her life completely.

When I caught up with her again, Robyn explained that the healing she received from that experience sent her on a quest to explore other practices and processes by other mediums, energy healers and holistic practitioners. "Karen, without a doubt, they all said so many of the same things. It was uncanny...and they all told me that I would be talking with teachers and healers from around the world, on my own show."

"Wow!" I said reenergized for the first time in days. "Well, I want to help you."

I revealed to Robyn my story. Why I had come to Discovery. My vision for the network and why this particular project for Oprah had been so important to me.

"Let me send you my pitch presentation."

A few hours later Robyn called me back. "OH-MY-GODD...." Were her first words to me. Her voice was choked up...was she crying? "Karen, the idea is amazing, your vision, wow, huge. But did you happen to notice the name of your presentation...the file name?"

I was lost. "I think it was something super creative like 'MY DECK?'" I said, really not following.

"Karen, the exact name of the file was 'MY DECK 11.17.2015.' 11.17 was my father's birthday. 11.17 is the name of my upcoming production company."

Well, hello Universe! Talk about a sign!!!

From that day forward, Robyn and I locked arms both in soul and in spirit. Our new adventure together had begun.

Two Soul Sisters on a Seeker's Mission

Meeting Robyn was the reason for the Oprah thing.

Here is her story.

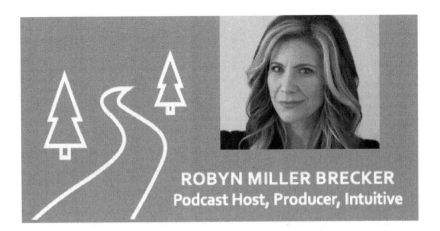

ROBYN MILLER BRECKER
Podcast Host, Producer, Intuitive

I have always moved through life trusting a "feeling." I didn't know that "feeling" was my intuition. In addition, I've always heard this inner voice talking to me... I assumed everyone had it -- and listened to it. I have since found out that almost everyone I know has it, but *not* everyone listens to it!

It wasn't until my late twenties that I understood that this inner voice was my soul, as well as Spirit, guiding me on this life's journey. A path that I created before I came into this lifetime.

For almost 20 years I worked for Oprah Winfrey, collaborating with some of the most brilliant thought leaders of our time. They helped me understand the power that we all hold within ourselves. They put a name to that "feeling".

In 2018, I felt like my soul was "dying." It was becoming increasingly harder to get out of bed and to sit through meetings. This feeling didn't just come out of the blue. It had been building within me for several years, but I couldn't understand why. I loved my husband and daughter; I had a solid support system. I had a sought-after-job with one of the most inspiring and powerful people in the world. What was this deep, inner longing for an alternate plan?

The fire that had always kept me motivated and smiling... was flaming out.

I felt lost, but I couldn't admit that to anyone except my husband and my sister. I didn't know what to do, and being the "responsible" person that I am, I didn't feel I could just quit my job without a plan. I also think I had Ego wrapped up in this — not just the actual job or who I worked for, but the not knowing of what would be next. What would I say to people? I felt trapped. I was sticking this job out until I had some sort of "aha" moment or a new plan.

And then... something happened!

On April 22, 2018, my 43rd birthday, the first of what would be a series of spiritual synchronicities began. I unexpectedly met up with a psychic who gave me some promising news. She said, "You do something really rare right now. You've been successful at whatever this is, BUT..." and then she pointed to the next column of Tarot cards and continued," ...this next thing you're going to do is going to be even more successful and aligned with your soul's purpose — your purpose for being here. And it's going to make you very noticed. Like famous."

I'm thinking...umm. Ok?!

She then went on to say that I will feel like things are aligned and on purpose when this next chapter starts. She also said that this will all take about a year to a year and a half to happen. "Don't quit your job tomorrow," she said, "but, I think you'll be done with your current job by the end of this year and then you'll be working on this next "thing" in 2019. February and March will be months of making things happen and then April/May things will come together quickly. This new chapter will be in full force by 2020."

After that reading, I felt mildly hopeful, but also a tad skeptical only because I didn't know the validity of that psychic.

Then, that same week, I had scheduled a reading with my dear friend, Lisa Nitin, who is a Spiritual Medium. I thought maybe my dad or my Spirit Team would have some guidance for me. Well, what happened blew me away.

Lisa not only reiterated everything that the psychic (who she didn't know!) said, she took it one step further.

When we started the session, Lisa said to me, "What are you working on right now?

I answered, "Nothing unusual."

Lisa insisted, "They're telling me you're doing SOMETHING different." Nothing came to mind.

I said, "That's why I'm here. I AM LOST."

Then Lisa said, "Please tell me what you are working on. They are saying that you are working on something that is going to lead to what you're really supposed to be doing with your life."

I said, "Well I'm writing an article that I'm calling "The Night A Medium Changed My Life"?

Her eyes widened and she screamed, "YES!!!!!! That's IT! That article is going to lead to other things...more articles or books or a show. And they are telling me that YOU ARE A MEDIUM. You can do this. You should be reading people."

I didn't even know what to say.

Lisa urged, "Promise me you'll at least take a class. I don't care if it's my class or another class, but take a class and see. It will help you with your writing. As I said, this is going to lead to articles or books or a show — this is IT. THIS is your next chapter. You're going to help awaken people this way."

HALLELUJAH!!!! I received the guidance that I needed!!! I have to say I was elated. I felt different. I felt awake. I felt relieved. Could this be what I'm meant to do? Could this fulfill my soul?

I wasn't exactly sure where it would all lead, but it gave me hope and direction.

Then after that there was even more. Over the next several months, out of nowhere, I was hooked up with a Shaman, another Psychic, an Astrologer and more. They didn't know me and they didn't know one another -- and they ALL said the SAME thing!! I was to start my own show and digital platform by 2020. The more I heard it, the more confident I became.

I began talking "as if" amongst my colleagues at work. "As if" I was going to have my own show, "as if" the next chapter had already begun. In one such meeting, I was with Karen. I was talking about my upcoming article, "The Night A Medium Changed My Life" that was going to post on Oprah.com. To my surprise, the people in the meeting were extremely interested in talking about Mediums, but we had to focus on the meeting at hand. I said, "don't worry, we'll talk much more about it on my show."

The whole room fell silent. I'm sure they were thinking, "what the heck is that woman, who works for Oprah, talking about?"

We got back to the meeting at hand.

Afterwards, Karen called me. She said, "Robyn, what show were you talking about in that meeting?"

I told Karen about my spiritual synchronicities over those past few months and what I was working towards. She said, "Count me in!"

A partnership was born.

I continued telling everyone and anyone what I was brewing, and I even spoke to my boss. Several months later there was a reorganization at my company and I was laid off. And, as the psychic and all of my other spiritual teachers and healers had predicted, I was done with my job at OWN by January 1, 2019.

I know this sounds weird, but for me, it was the best news ever!

I was given a severance package and 1117 Productions was established. *Seeking with Robyn* has become a reality. I chose to trust and love the Universe -- and myself, instead of clinging to what was familiar and "safe". For the first time in many years, I feel alive and aligned with my soul's purpose and excited for all that's to come!

Speaking Your Truth

I wanted to share that full story with you, because it totally changed my path. And the same thing can happen to you.

Robyn began creating her reality the minute she began speaking her truth with the words of her vision out loud. She got me and everyone on our conference call excited when she told us about her TV show. Think about what would have happened if she hadn't shared her dream with me. We would have missed out on an opportunity to pool our resources and create our vision of an even broader, far reaching idea than we would have accomplished with Discovery.

We were now looking at creating a vision together of content and programming that we know we are meant to design and launch as a team!

Speaking your truth is what activates your dreams; it is the most important step in bringing your dreams to your door.

Let me show you how.

LIFEMAPPING EXPLORATION #10 – Part 2

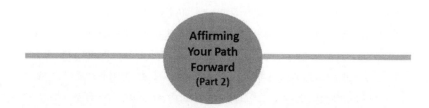

This is the final Lifemapping exploration. It is the easiest, but by far, the most powerful.

In this experience, it is you who will be writing the final "Soulfirmation" by taking your newly recalibrated "I am statements" and putting them together into your own uniquely personalized, affirming expression of your life's purpose.

The steps are simple.

- Step 1: **Create Your Personalized Soul-firmation**: Take all of your newly created, positive action statements from your prior exercise on p. ## and place them together on the following page. If you can, print or write them out so you can place them in a place you can see every day.

- Step 2: **Step Up to The Manifestation Microphone**: This is the most important part. As you absorb the amazing statement that you have compiled about your soul's purpose...it is important to read the words OUTLOUD. While it may feel strange at first to speak these statements, it is the best way to give them actionable, manifestation POWER. And, if you can share these words with someone else, it doubles the power...because it engages another in your positive energy flow. This is precisely how prayer works…. and if you are not a religious believer, think of this as a way of boosting the light and voice of your affirmation. As you do this exercise…imagine yourself in front of an actual microphone where your angels, soul guides (on this planet and beyond) are there in your audience, cheering you on.

- **Steps 3: Establish Your Practice:** I'm sharing mine on the next page so you can get a sense of the beautiful poetry that comes from activating these pure statements of your inner truth. I try to re-read mine daily.

  This manifestation mantra can be used in your daily practice:

  1. Sleep Routine: When you wake up in the morning and before you go to bed: Think of this as your seedling to start your day grounded to your truth, and as the last thought in your subconscious that your mind can marinate on as it slumbers.
  2. Tape it to your bathroom mirror: This will enable you to fill your mind with positivity when you brush your teeth, blow dry your hair and shave.
  3. Record it: Play it as your daily meditation or in the car or headphones as you drive to work.

OK, here's the backdrop for you to use for your dream vision. This is your own, personal, Soulfirmation, customized just for you!

MY LIFEMAP SOULFIMATION: Affirming My Purpose

_____
_____
_____
_____
_____
_____
_____
_____
_____
_____
_____
_____
_____
_____
_____
_____
_____
_____
_____
_____
_____

As always, here's mine to share with you.

MY LIFEMAP SOULFIMATION: Affirming My Purpose

I am here to teach others how to be courageous and strong.
I am here to show others how to believe in themselves and not give up.
I am here to show others how to be an explorer and dreamer.
I am accepting and proud of myself.
I am at ease and confident in my success.
I am unafraid and uninfluenced by other's options or judgements.
I am here to be a storyteller.
I am here to be a teacher.
I am here to be a seeker.
I am wise and always know what to do.
I know I was born to follow my talents and desires and when I do it will bring me success.
I am worthy of unconditional love from myself and others.
I am here to share my talents as a writer & creator.
I am here to inspire people and elevate their energy.
I am here to share my spiritual ideas with others.
I let go of the need to control the outcome.
I am more than enough. I was born to do this!
I have accumulated wisdom and skills I need to succeed.

Well done! How does it feel? You have gone the distance. You have done the work. You now have a vision of where you've been, where you are, and where you want to go from here.

As you reflect upon your beautifully written affirmation, I invite you to review some of the key things that we have learned together in this chapter, and reflect how you can apply them to your own vision.

These are really powerful tools, my friends.

1. **SEE IT + BELIEVE IT = ALLOW IT.** That's the formula of manifestation. So, in my story, I could see what I wanted to create, but the believing and allowing took some big-time work. And it wasn't until I truly let go that the Oprah opportunity came through.

    *   What is it that you see that you want for yourself? Is it the job, the relationship, the new life living in a whole new place?
    *   Can you identify the ways you might be disallowing yourself from getting what you want by holding on too tight to it or NOT being in the here and now just yet?

2. **Reactivate & Re-callibrate** – In my case, I had to do some work on my beliefs before I could get myself to a place of believing enough in my own self to be worthy of my dream. Doing the affirmations to reactivate self-love and recalibrate the fear into positives, went a long way to helping reshape my self-love.

    *   What are the purpose affirmations that can help you believe in your own self-worth?

- What does your life map tell you that your dream is? Do you believe in it?
- Are there ways of rewording your affirmations to help you activate where you want to go from here?

3. **Have a mind that is open to everything and attached to nothing.** To allow it, you have to let it go. Because, yeah, you guessed it- the universe always has bigger plans for you than you can ever imagine.

Let's finish our work with some powerful thoughts from the great positive thinker, writer, pastor, mentor, manifester and Master Mind creator, Rev. Jack Boland.

How to Change Your World

Whatever your state of mind, it is so powerful that it cannot be hidden from the world. What you have confidence in will come to you – be it good or bad. It will come to you!

There is no power on this earth that will keep it from coming. Your silent command will be obeyed. All that is required is that you really believe and have no doubt. Our thoughts and feelings reach out into life to touch, to grasp, to catch hold of and then bring back that which we believe in.

If you don't like your world, change the thoughts and feelings that are creating it. Our personal world is composed of what our thoughts bring to us. It is absolutely incredible how the mind works. That is why it is said that "what the mind of man can conceive and believe, it can achieve."

—Rev. Jack Boland

SOUL GOODY BAG

Here are some resources mentioned in this chapter for you for further exploration:

- **Robyn Miller Brecker:** Robyn is an Emmy® award winning producer and leader in content development. For 20 years she worked for Oprah Winfrey, collaborating with some of the most brilliant thought leaders of our time to create programming that has impacted millions. Prior to her time with Ms. Winfrey, she was part of the team that launched the children's television network, Noggin, and also lived out some of her green slime dreams at Nickelodeon. She has always been at the forefront of combining wisdom, technology and storytelling to inspire and bring like-minded people together. After a series of spiritual synchronicities in 2018, Robyn's life was transformed and "Seeking with Robyn" was imagined. She even considers herself an intuitive and a Spiritual Medium in the making! In March 2020, she launched her YouTube show, "Seeking with Robyn" and in August 2020 she made the show available as a podcast, on all podcast platforms. For more about Robyn check out her website: seekingwithrobyn.com

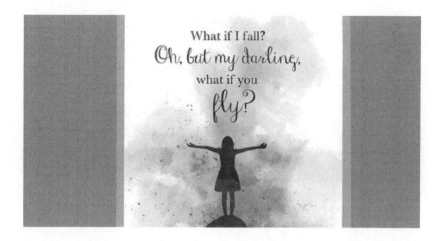

What if I fall?
Oh, but my darling,
what if you
fly?

CHAPTER 12

MAKING YOUR VISION COME TRUE: YOUR SOUL TOOLBOX

You know that big map in the airport or in the shopping mall that is marked with a big arrow that says, "you are here"? Well, my dearest darling, this is where you are now on your Life Map. And what a long way you have come!

When we began this journey in Chapter One, we came together with the intention of creating a map for you to better understand your life's purpose, why you are here, and remind you of the tools you have been given as you chart your path though this incarnation of life.

I hope some of these exercises have given you insight into the marvelous, creation that you are. Each and every one of us has within the seed to blossom into that which we intended to give the world - which is the precious gift of ourselves. And yet, how often do we downplay our greatness, and not see the amazing treasure that we are?

As you have taken stock of your life's milestones and key moments, and taken time to identify and recalibrate your relationships with love and fear, I hope that you are now better able to see the lessons that they have given you. You can use these lessons to build the foundation of the next phase of your life. This is your life school, your sandbox. You have always been, and will always be free to see, and do whatever you want with it.

But now you can chart the next epic part of your journey from a place of understanding and do it with inspiration and intention. Now you have come to the place on your life map where you get to truly be the captain of your own ship and chart the course for where you want to go.

One of the reasons that I love the cover of my book is that it's such a fitting symbol for the "where to go from here" question, and for this last chapter in particular. The little girl is looking at the unpaved road in front of her. It's as if she's suddenly stopped to catch her breath. Although we can't see her face, she seems to exude forceful determination, defiance perhaps, as she looks ahead, with hands on her hips and the wind blowing in her hair.

And so is my vision for you. I can't see your face at this very moment. However, it is my hope that you now have a sense of where you've come from, with a deeper understanding of who you are. This deep understanding of self will enable you to move forward with that same determination towards the next part of your journey.

Your dreams are never stagnate or complete; they are always evolving.

This chapter is all about the "moving forward." Now that your vision is complete, I'll share some tools that can help make your dream a reality. Simple practices that will keep your light shining on your plans and future outcomes, and keep the momentum for playing them forward.

You have taken the hero's journey. You know who you are. You know the roots of your loves and your fears. You know why you are here and have some ideas for what you want to do. Now it is about taking everything to the next level.

So, how do you make your vision come true?

Here you can learn how to activate your life map using 4 simple tools that will continue to amplify your vision so it can breathe, morph, grow and freely evolve as you venture down your highway.

Here we'll take the manifestation formula of SEE/BELIEVE/ALLOW/MANIFEST and apply it in a slightly different way. *By using your intuition, following your inspiration, activating your intention and harnessing your imagination, you will be able to move forward knowing that you can acquire and achieve, and continue to let your life map evolve.*

Are you ready to rumble with the universe?

Paving Your Road Forward: Following Your Bliss

Author and theologian, Joseph Campbell, is perhaps best known for coining the phrase "follow your bliss." The adage was embraced by the New Age movement in the early eighties, inspiring many books and even movies that provoked millions to ask themselves to do the thing that inspired happiness from the whisperings of their soul. Even the great filmmaker George Lucas, deemed Joseph Campbell "my Yoda" claiming he inspired the storyline of the "Star Wars" series.

Among his many mythological and aspirational writings, Campbell once said, "We must be willing to let go of the life we planned so as to have the life that is waiting for us." He also said, "The cave your fear to enter, holds the treasure that you seek."

Sounds like Yoda to me.

When I listened to Joseph Campbell being interviewed for the first time, it was as if he was speaking to my soul. I was in my mid-twenties, sorting through my own personal narrative, trying to carve out the path to a career that I could not quite envision, yearning to figure out how I could possibly fit in. Campbell's epic question teed up an idea that I'd never seriously considered.

"What is it that makes you happy?" he asked during the now famous PBS Special with Bill Moyers, "Not excited, not just thrilled, but deeply happy?" It seemed like such a simple question. But deep happiness seemed at odds with the concept of prosperity and success. Wasn't it all about the hard work, challenge, competition, struggle, sacrifice and earning of accomplishment? Happiness seemed...well, too simple.

Exactly.

"Stay with that," Campbell said, "No matter what people tell you. This is what is called 'following your bliss.'" Bliss, in Campbells view, was a simple framing of happiness...those tranquil moments in time that feel deeply fulfilling, meaning-ful and real. But bliss just wasn't a word that my high school guidance counselor had ever used. And it certainly wasn't how corporations were compensating their employees.

And next I heard the big shebang. The thing that lit my mind on fire. Campbell said this:

"If you follow your bliss, you put yourself on a kind of track that has been there all the while waiting for you, and

then the life you ought to be living is the one you are living. Follow your bliss and don't be afraid. If you follow your bliss, doors will open for you that wouldn't have opened for anyone else."

This was like having the holy grail hiding in plain sight.

Bliss doesn't have to be a "big," over the moon, in-love-kinda-thing. Bliss is not a perpetual state of being. Bliss is a beacon. It's like a delicious smell or our favorite song on the radio. It fills you. It makes you feel good. When you think of it, a light illuminate. You smile. It tugs to your attention. It makes you go deeper, think longer. You linger. You savor.

Bliss is joy. Bliss is peace. Bliss is being. Bliss and our souls are one.

Bliss is the compass of your LifeMap. Bliss is your GPS for where you go from here.

Your Blisstopia

Here's the thing that gets people nervous about "taking the risk of their bliss". I know it may be scary to think that knitting, going to garage sales, or gardening could be your bliss, when outwardly, you know there's no potential way that these passion projects could pay your bills right now. But I encourage you to begin making the time to nurture these fantasies every possible chance you get. They may not be your *sole-source* of what will fill up your bank account, but it will be your *soul-source* of what fills up your spirit.

Your Blisstopia is ever evolving... but like your soul's purpose, it was born within you.

In our last chapter, we identified your personal brand of blisstopia when we translated all of your life experiences into one soul-affirming statement. And now that you have that soul-ful reflection of who you are, here's where you'll access the tools to help your nurture that thing, idea, dream, or wish and plant it in a pot of possibility.

Life is, in fact, about enjoying the journey. But having a destination is fun too.

So, let's go take a ride on the bliss train.

How to Become a Sorcerer

Bliss tends to show up in places of ease, beauty, rest, openness and appreciation. It is like the magic wand of your fairy godmother, who can grant you your highest wish and make your dreams come true.

Sounds like a fairy tale? It's not. And you don't need your fairy godmother or a magic wand to get you stuff. You have the power already inside you.

Remember in the movie the Wizard of Oz, when Dorothy's little dog peaks behind the curtain, and reveals the Wizard is not a fierce, fire-breathing magician, but just a mild-mannered traveling salesman from the mid-west? After the initial disappointment of discovering that he wasn't who they thought he was when he set them off on the dangerous quest to bring back the witch's broom, Dorothy and her companions learn that their adventures had taught them valuable lessons using skills and talents that they had all along.

The Tinman wanted a heart, but discovered he already had one by showing the love he had for his friends as he helped them navigate their dangerous journey. The scarecrow longed for a brain, but showed he already had one by helping his friends calculate their escape from the prison of the wicked witch. The lion, who yearned for courage, discovered he was already brave by facing the wrath of the witch's evil army. And then Dorothy, once desperate to leave home and now longing to find her way back, learns she's always had the power to get there right from the beginning, with her red ruby slippers.

We are all born with our magical superpowers within us... we just have to learn how to use them.

In his books, Wayne Dyer spoke endlessly about the powers of Inspiration, Intuition, Intention and imagination as being an omniscient force that propels and manages the universe. He also ascribed our own power as "sorcerers," or "those who live from a place connected to their source, a oneness with our own true divine selves, who can activate love, and release ego are those who can generate virtually anything that they want to be, have or desire.

How does this translate your beautiful **Purpose Affirmation Statement into** your reality?

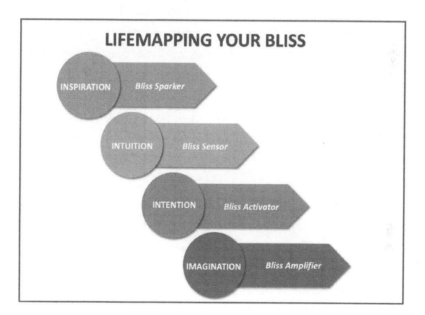

The answer is simple- you utilize your 4 Bliss power tools. Your Four "I's"

1. Your Bliss Sparker - INSPIRATION
2. Your Bliss Sensor - INTUITION
3. Your Bliss Activator - INTENTION
4. Your Bliss Amplifier - INTENTION

You've heard of them, right?

If you're like me...you probably LOVE the potential behind those four words... they feel creative, energetic, powerful. OF COURSE THEY DO! Because we've all experienced little morsels of their magic... a little twinge of their fairy dust in our midst.

But to be real, the Four "I's" have never really gotten the collective credibility they deserve. In the hard and fast, factual, show-me-the-money world, intuition, inspiration, intention, and imagination are often deemed as soft, self-help idioms; intangible and immeasurable. But alas, those poor, practical realists! Living in the so-called real world, where the "I's represent the land of the sentimentalists – those Pollyanna's who believe in fairy tales?

Well yeah!

Remember when Cinderella's Fairly Godmother came to help put her package together to go to the ball, and Cinderella just couldn't get her head around the idea? She was skeptical about the pumpkin becoming the stagecoach, and the mouse becoming the driver. I mean who wouldn't be, right? It wasn't "sensible."

But that's when the Fairy Godmother spoke up for dreamers everywhere when she said:

"The sensible people will say Fol-de-rol and fiddle dee dee and fiddley faddley foodle all the dreamers in the world are dizzy in the noodle."

"And aren't they?" asked Cinderella. "Not always," said her fairy godmother. "The world is full of zanies and fools who don't believe in sensible rules and won't believe what sensible people say... and because these daft and dewy-eyed dopes keep building up impossible hopes, impossible things are happening every day!"

How I loved those days when my innocent young mind didn't question the possibilities of those "far-fetched" happy endings for Dorothy and Cinderella. Do you remember when you still believed in so called "fairy tales?"

How sad for those that don't understand the true magical powers of our sixth senses! For those who know how to utilize this co-creative dance with destiny, the four "i's" are among the most powerful tools in the universe. They are the source from which all creation comes from.

So, no surprises here. Inspiration, intuition, intention and imagination are your compadres on your ongoing Lifemapping journey.

So, let's put them to work for you.

Befriending Your Blissful Bestie's

Let's begin sharpening your ninja skills around the 4 "I's" and hook you up with tools you can use to till your bliss garden blossoms. As you review each of these tools, keep your "AFFIRMING MY PURPOSE" vision statement within reach. And note where each of these tools trigger ideas that further flesh out your vision.

1. Inspiration: Your Bliss "Sparker":

> *"There is a voice in the universe entreating us to remember our purpose, our reason for being here now in this world of impermanence. The voice whispers, shouts and sings to us that this experience – of being in form in space and time – has meaning. That voice belongs to inspiration, which is within each and every one of us."*
>
> —Wayne Dyer -Inspiration, Your Ultimate Calling (p.3)

Inspiration has got to be one of my favorite words. Inspiration is a feeling of lightness...possibility...creation...anticipation. It's that sudden realization or knowingness from somewhere out of the blue. It's a spark of an idea, a thought, a sense of joyful recognition. An 'aha" moment seemingly coming from out of nowhere. Inspiration is a wink from the universe.

I think of the word *inspiration* as meaning "being in-spirit" or connected to the essence of who were really are...our source. And indeed, at its root, to "inspire" means "to bring to life" or "to give breath to." What better place to begin with anything we do?

Inspiration is the first of the four "I's" because it is that spark that ignites us from the outside. It is a serendipitous force. You might be in the shower, you might be looking at a beautiful landscape, you might be just quietly listening to music, when that feeling taps on your shoulder. Most often you are in a place of receiving or appreciation...a state of mind that is not concentrating on creating, when inspiration catches you off guard. That's when the idea that you have been searching for, the solution you have been seeking, suddenly comes and sits beside you.

What are some of the things that have inspired you that you know have had an impact on you along the way? Was it a movie? A book? A person? A place? A mentor? A beautiful landscape? All of these things?

As you continue to evolve and add to your LifeMap, inspiration will always be one of your best friends. It is the muse that knows your heart's desires and will continue to summon more delights from the universe to add sparkle to your dreams, wishes and desires. Inspiration is your dream sensor, and your co-creator. Inspiration will flutter to you like a butterfly on the wings of possibility.

Bliss "Sparkers": Tools for Developing Your Inspiration:

Your Bliss Sparkers are the experiences that come from "outside" of you that can be conduits, triggers or backdrops for inspirational thoughts and ideas to appear.

I would softly suggest, whenever possible, that you experience these Bliss Sparkers solo...for the least possible distraction to be able to experience and receive your messages fully.

1. **Heed the Call of Nature:** Best way I know (which is why it is number one) to get inspired. Drinking in the beauty of nature and breathing in the magic of the earth's landscape will bring your brain and body to a place of quiet openness and receptivity for your intuition to arrive.

2. **Lock Yourself in the Bathroom:** One of the best ways to let your brain relax and ease into a good

inspirational idea is a good warm soak or shower...and I do believe that ions in the water help massage our "third eye" also known as the pituitary gland, which is our receptor of our inspired thoughts and insights.

3. **Hit the Open Road:** There's something about the lull of a long drive and the fact that we can turn off the world inside our car if we so choose. It can be a portal for muffling out the world's noise and turning up the radio to dedicate time to open up to the unseen language of our thoughts.

4. **Become a Drifter:** There's nothing better to get you feeling more aligned than floating in a gentle pool or ocean waves and looking up at the sky. This can also apply to drifting on a raft on a lake, sitting in a boat, floating downstream in a canoe...or just kicking back in a backyard pool or jacuzzi. There's just something about letting go and drifting to where the water takes you, that brings us back to resting in receiving mode, where inspiration is cleared to pay a visit.

5. **Change It Up:** Taking off to explore a nearby town or place that you've never visited, jumping on a train to watch the world go by, or just rearranging the furniture in your bedroom can offer a signal to the universe that you are ready and open for change or a new perspective. Visit a Museum, monument or library to glean inspiration from the artists, creators and change makers from the past to summon their magic of artistry, creativity and impact on the present.

6. **Get Centered:** Even if you swear you can't do it.... there are many different approaches (and benefits), of regular mindfulness practice. Some say just ten minutes of mediation can equate to 44 minutes of sleep, not to mention help you reconnect to the voice of your own soul. There are many great meditation apps now that you can download and use for free.

7. **Catch Your Breath:** Breath work is quickly becoming my latest go-to for affirming all the needs of my mind, body and spirit. I would challenge you, as you read this now, to monitor your breathing, just for a minute. Are your breaths shallow, and infrequent? I had to learn how to fill my lungs and take deep, nourishing breaths...and when I did...ah...how my brainwaves kicked in! Besides enhancing your inspiration, there are health benefits from deep breathing exercises that include reducing stress levels in your body, lowering blood pressure, reducing depression, helping manage chronic pain, and helping regulate your body's reaction to stress and fatigue.

8. **Take Five:** Why has the art of resting become such a luxury? Taking time to shut off your brain during the day, even for 20 minutes has been proven to promote attention, boost memory and yeah, open yourself up to inspired moments. And if you really want a mental massage, try donning your headphones and immerse yourself in the magical music tones of the Solfeggio Frequencies. The ancient sound frequencies have been integrated into blissful meditative melodies that can promote relaxation and recalibration to put your mind in inspiration mode.

9. **Soothe Your Nerves:** Today there are more economical choices than ever to integrate nourishing massage or Reiki treatment into your routine. Medical research shows that even an occasional session can help reduce stress, physical pain and fatigue, and also improve immunity, sleep, and emotional balance.

10. **Do a Digital Detox:** Take a break from your devices even if it's just a few hours on a weekend to escape and to have some deep alone time with your best friends, "me, myself and I" to enjoy the sounds, and inspirational power of silence.

2. Intuition: Your Bliss "Sensor"

"There is a universal, intelligent life force that exists within everyone and everything. It resides within each one of us as a deep wisdom, an inner knowing. We can access this wonderful source of knowledge and wisdom through our intuition, and inner sense that tells us what feels right and true for us at any given moment."

—Shakti Gawain
Developing Intuition:
Developing Guidance for Daily Life

Intuition is the ability to understand something immediately and inwardly, without the need for conscious reasoning. It's a thing that one knows from an instinctive feeling, a knowingness that may not necessarily be explained, or logical. A "mother's intuition" is that 6th sense when she knows there's a problem with her child, or a cop's "hunch" when there's trouble afoot. Intuition is an instinct...something you just know from personal experience. It's a deep awareness that you might not be able to readily explain. An inward GPS that can help you make judgements when there are no rulebooks to follow.

Intuition speaks with a quiet voice...which is why we often overlook it. But it is also a voice that will not be silent...and it can be relentless...because it is the voice of our greatest truths. I like to think of Intuition as those inner nudges from your soul. And your soul is miserable if it is ignored or told what it cannot do.

Listen if it beckons you in a certain direction. It will never lead you astray.

Step 2: Your Bliss "Sensor": Tools for to Developing Your Intuition:

Your Bliss Sensors are the tools of your inner guidance... they live "inside" of you and are the barometers of your intuitive guidance system... these can be thoughts, feelings, emotions, and interpretations of messages that utilize your intuitive instincts that can spark a new insight, understanding or feeling of clarity about your LifeMap path.

Here are a few ideas to help you develop and use your intuition sensors to support you on your Lifemapping journey.

Bliss Sensors: Tools for Developing Your Intuition:

1. **Trust Your Vibes:** We were given our bodily senses to help us safely navigate our way through the world... and all of them contribute to utilizing our most important sense of all, our 6th sense, our gut, our

instinct, our intuition. Our Intuition helps us read the energy in a room or the disguised feelings others might be having about us. It is that unseen knowingness, that "feeling," that may be indistinguishable with our outside bodily feelers, that can sense the invisible. The more we trust it, the more it will be our most valued ally.

2. **Work Your Clair's:** The Clair senses are types of "psychic" abilities that correspond with the five senses of seeing, hearing, feeling, smelling and tasting. Tapping into the 5 "spiritual" Clair's is another way of accessing the fourth dimensional energy of the unseen, which is nonetheless, just as real.

   i.   Clairvoyance means clear seeing.
   ii. Clairaudience means clear hearing.
   iii. Clairsentience means clear feeling.
   iv. Clairalience means clear smelling.
   v.   Clairgustance means clear tasting.
   vi. Claircognizance means clear knowing.

   There are many credible resources for developing your Clair senses, that can provide you with a whole new layer of intuitive guidance. For more on understanding your intuitive gifts and your clair senses, check out Rebecca Rosen's book "Awaken the Spirit Within."

3. **Get Carded:** Tarot and Angel cards are popular tools that can prompt intuitive messages. Traditionally, they are interpreted by card readers who have been trained to understand the specific meanings of each

card, and many have their own methodology for providing readings. You may also choose your own deck, and use it as a source for connecting to your angels and guides to ask them to provide their own messages for you.

4. **Channel a Free-Write**: I love to spend a few minutes after meditation tapping into my "inner/higher self" to offer a few dedicated minutes for my soul to speak. This can be in the form of asking about a specific question, or just allowing what "comes" to go from thought to paper. Some of my most intimate, loving words have been written to me from that higher state and have helped me develop my intuition.

5. **Follow Your Dreams:** The hours we spend with our conscious mind shut off, offers us unbounded time to explore the deep, limitless, mysterious recesses of our subconscious. According to astrologer and dream expert Dr. Michael Lennox, "The unconscious mind expresses itself in symbols, and these symbols form a language of their own. When I listen to someone describe a dream, I hear it as a story told in this symbolic language." According to Michael, if we offer the intention to remember our dreams before we go to bed, we will often remember them when we wake up...and if we quickly write them down, we have a magical opportunity to discover deep messages about ourselves. Michael's book, Dream Sight: A Dictionary and Guide for Interpreting Any Dream, is one of two books that he's written on the subject that can help you decipher the many stories from your slumber.

6. **Read the Signs:** Back in chapter XX – we explored how to look for signs from our departed loved ones and guides, as a way of affirming their support or presence with us as we navigate our path. So too, as we are looking to affirm our own decisions, questions and ideas with our own intuition, we can ask for specific signs from the universe to help validate that we are going in the right direction. We can ask for any kind of sign...a visit from a spirit animal, a certain song coming on the radio, a connection to a person or piece of information that affirms our intuition, is a wonderful game to play for both clarity and validation.

7. **Follow the Stars:** Learning more about your birth chart and numerology is another path for validating not only your soul's purpose, but to do check-ins on the ongoing planetary influences on your life. According to our friend Stevie Calista, who we met in Chapter X, a birth chart reading is "a blueprint for each person. It helps us see what gifts and challenges we came into this life with and how we can use them. It shows us how our head and heart speak to each other." If that's not a place to follow intuition, what is? For more about Stevie's readings, visit farmhousemoon.com.

8. **Explore Your Past Lives:** Past life regression therapy can be an enlightening and life-changing way to use the past to open your insights into the future. According to Spiritual Development Coach and Past Life Regressionist Michelle Brock, who we met in chapter X, "Past life regression is a chance to not just

believe or have faith that there is a greater design and purpose to our existence, it is a chance to experience it directly. It can help you to know more about who you are, why you are here, and even to discover what your unique, divine purpose is in life." Talk about a way to intimately and intuitively get to know your eternal soul!!! Michelle can be reached here. https://michelle-brock.com/about-michelle-brock/

3. Intention: Your Bliss "Activator":

Intent is a force that exists in the universe. When sorcerers (those who live of the Source) beckon intent, it comes to them and sets up the path for attainment, which means that sorcerers always accomplish what they set out to do.

—Carlos Castandeda

There is within all of us an inner whisper that intends for us to express ourselves. That something is your soul telling you that there is something you need to do and share with the world...we know, through our earlier work together that this is the voice of love, your purpose, of all that you have intended to do with this lifetime. That silent inner knowing will never leave you alone. This is the voice of your intention...that desirous, ravenous, passionate, willful part of you that motivates you to get it done. To do what it is that you have come to do.

I like to think of intention as your inner 5-year-old, that really, really wants that new toy...and will stop at nothing, I mean nothing, to get it.

The intention of your inner child still lives...we just need to channel it. Intention isn't something that we do; it's an energy we attract.

Your Bliss Activators are those desires percolating through your soul that are aching to activate...to manifest, to become reality. They are the drivers of your soul bus.

Here are a few ideas for activating your intentions.

Bliss Activators: Ways to Use the Power of Intentions

1. **Start with one thing** – Remember when we talked about how the journey of a thousand miles begins with a single step? If Lifemapping has opened up a big idea or dream for you, that is tremendous! And if you are still contouring the first draft of your vision sketch, that's amazing too. As the pixy dust is the first step to flying, remember that this isn't about orchestrating the entire symphony. Pick one song, one instrument, even one note to focus on, and see where it takes you. It's not about "*what*" you do, it's about the *intention energy* that you bring to it.

2. **Watch your words** – This was an early lesson handed down to me from my mother from Louise Hay. There is nothing more powerful than the spoken word. And "**how**" you say it, it as important as "**what**" you say. Replace words like "should," and "don't" with "could" and "can" and you immediately shift the energy in your favor. Instead of saying "I should have a job," or "I don't have a partner" use sentences like "I could have a job," or "I can have a partner" and your whole point of attraction changes.

3. **Make It a Bedtime Story** –Remember when you were a child and you read a bedtime story and said your evening prayers? Why as we grow older, do so many of us lose sight of the power we have to realign our thoughts as we head off into slumber? How many times do we waste our last precious hours of the day thinking about our mistakes, regrets, grievances, losses, instead of taking a gratitude inventory on everything you have and wish for? Whether you believe in God, Source, a higher power, or the power of yourself, purposing time for your bedtime ritual to "imbed" your desires for what you will focus on as you sleep, knowing there is no better way to utilize your 6-8 hours of slumber than to let your subconscious mind percolate on your intentions.

4. **Avoid low energy people** – You know who they are. They're the ones with opinions. The ones who have your "best interests" at heart. They're the harkeners of so-called "reality," who can see all of the land-mines and pitfalls who want to be sure that you stay safe. These are the well-meaning ones who tell you why your intended dream or idea is dangerous for you. According to best-selling author Brene Brown, while we have to "reserve a seat" for both the critics and our own self-doubt" as we follow our dreams, "If you are not out there in the arena, getting your ass kicked," Brene adds, "I'm not interested in your feedback." Don't let the critics and the well-meaning naysayers get a vote, and remain committed to your intentions no matter what others say.

5. **Give your ego the heave ho** – This is probably the toughest one to officially manage, because our fear-based self loves to point out all the reasons why our dreams and desires should challenge us. Whenever you sense that your inner chatter has become more about the "why's" of all of the reasons standing in your way, try to catch yourself and flip your ego on its head. Ask yourself, "Why not?" and replay the reasons that you can come up with. Use your list of "I am's" to help remind you of all of the love-based strengths that you already have in your soul's DNA... and know that you only have to focus on a fraction of that goodness for positive manifestation to come your way.

6. **Put them in Writing** – Whether you create them as a digital screen saver, or post them on your bathroom mirror, creating a visual space gives our intentions the front row in our day. Like brushing your teeth, or making your morning pot of coffee, this is the way you continue to give your subconscious mind an affirmation "work-out"- by integrating them into a habitual visualization that becomes part of your daily routine.

7. **Create a sacred space** – Speaking of daily rituals, setting up a dedicated nook, shelf, altar, or Zen garden, is another way to create a venue in which to routinely affirm your intentions. For some beautiful examples on how to set up sacred spaces and simple spiritual practices, check out "The Spirit Almanac, A Modern Guide to Ancient Self Care," where Mind Body Green authors, Emma Loewe and Lindsay Kellner, offer easy

tips for turning simple ceremonies for the mind, body and soul into self-care practices you can use every day.

8. **Just say yes** – invite the universe to surprise you with unexpected opportunities for discovery, by embracing new opportunities, and yes, even challenges when they come your way. You never know when a door can open to a brand-new world of people, places and experiences, until you dare to step out of your comfort zone.

9. **Ask "how can I serve?"** – by offering out the intention to help others, and taking the focus off of our own needs and desires, we can open up a place within ourselves for receiving, and potentially fill the void of what's missing in ourselves. I remember when my friend Grace, who was trying for years to conceive a child, became pregnant after releasing her focus on a baby, by first becoming a mom by adopting a dog from a shelter. Getting to a place of surrendering our own desire for outcome, to do for others, puts us in the energy-mode of giving love which then puts us in a place of receiving love as well.

10. **Reaffirm your I am's** – Whenever you feel like you're are losing ground with your intentions, go back to chapter x and re-read your "I am" statements, to remind yourself of the powerful soul you have come to be. Say them out loud, in front of the mirror if possible, and look yourself in the eye as you speak these powerful words of your inner truth. Tell yourself, and tell the world that THIS is the you that you

have INTENDED to come to be. You ARE, those embodiments of spirit. Visualize the brightness of your light, and know you ARE already these amazing qualities. External realities only represent a tiny fraction of the internal, eternal, spiritual being that you are.

11. **Release expectations of outcome** - Use positive mantras that keep your energy positive, like "Everything is easy for me," or "I am ready to receive (fill in the blank), or something even better." And then know and believe that, no matter what, the outcome will reflect your highest good.

12. **Know that the universe has your back** - You are a spiritual being having a human experience. You are a great and powerful co-creator of source. Let this translate to knowingness that your intention is riding an unseen wave of energy and there is nothing that you can't be, have or do.

4. Imagination: Your Bliss "Amplifier"

"The greatest gift you were ever given was the gift of your imagination. Within your magical inner realm, is the capacity to have all your wishes fulfilled. Here in your imagination is the greatest power that you will ever know. It is your domain for creating the life that you desire and the best part of it is that you are the monarch with all of the inherent powers to rule your world as you desire."

—Dr. Wayne W. Dyer, Wishes Fulfilled

Look around the room you are sitting in now. Virtually everything in front of you has been created from someone's imagination. How many of these things were even in existence twenty years ago? And how many of those creations, just one hundred years earlier, would have been considered crazy or impossible?

And so, it is for you, with absolutely anything you can envision in your own mind's eye.... anything within the realm of possibility. You were never given a dream without the power to make it so. And yet, that vision can seem tactically impossible and out of reach.

"I resent the limitations of my own imagination." Those are the words of Walt Disney, who created an empire around the idea of translating his ideas and making wishes come true. His vision for producing animated movie features brought his vision of entertaining the "child in all of us" to a new frontier. From the beginning, he searched for ways to make Disney innovative and different from other companies. It was Walter Disney's ambition to give his audience the very best, so the execution of his pioneering ideas was never left to chance. Dream. Believe. Dare. Do. That was his mantra. Disney also said, "If you can dream it, you can do it." Such a seemingly simple statement is another four-step program that contains the magic formula for making a vision, an idea, or a wish into a reality.

The definition of imagination is 'the action of forming new ideas, or images or concepts of external objects not present to the senses." The term **imagination** comes from the Latin verb imaginari **meaning** "to picture oneself." I like to think of imagination as transforming an image into reality.

Imagination is magical. Imagination is the act of conception with the infinite. It is a sorcerer's harnessing source used to intertwine the threads of inspiration, intuition, intention and weaving their golden transformative tapestry into the fabric of imagination.

Here are some ways that imagination can work for you.

Bliss Amplifier: Ways to Use the Power of Your Imagination

1. **Become an Imagineer** – Like Walt Disney's team of creators, the Imagineers, you too have the power to bring your imagination to life. Use whatever tools you choose to create and craft a place to draft and hold your vision. This can be in a notebook, on a bulletin board, in a Pinterest Page, or on a spreadsheet...wherever you can manipulate and rework your thoughts in a way that feels like ever organic and evolutionary vision of you. Be bold!

2. **Craft a 1 - 3-5 Year Envision Statement**–Play a little of the "life review" game in reverse. Imagine you are telling your story to your child or grandchild in the future. What did you do? Who did you meet? How did you feel? What was your contribution? What was your mantra? Be as specific with the details as you can, and hone in on how you felt during the journey of your experience. Have fun sharing how the vision evolved the first year, into the third year, into the 5th year and beyond.

3. **Act as if** – In every possible moment, experience the feeling that you have already achieved your vision, and "act as if" you are already living the life of your dreams. In Wayne Dyers' book, "Wishes Fulfilled," he talks about the importance of "thinking from the end" and embracing the feeling of a new situation

even though it isn't there yet. "By literally feeling the reality of the state that you seek," Wayne writes, "which is firmly in your imagination, you have the means of creating miracles." (p.102) Sounds like fun to me!

4. **Play the Movie in your Mind** – As we discovered in Chapter **3,** one of the most fun games you can play in your imagination is creating the "movie in your mind." So, what is your story? If Hollywood was going to produce a movie of your life, what would the highlights be? Where would your breakthrough moments come from? How would you want your story to inspire the other aspiring dreamers that are out there? Have fun with this vision and play around with the endings.

5. **Write your Bio** – This is a really fun exercise to really rewrite your resume in a whole new way. Knowing where you are today, what are the dream jobs that you wish to hold. Where will you work? What level of responsibility do you wish to hold? Are you running your own shop or are you part of an international corporation? Again, it's all about trying different roles on for size, and *feeling* how they fit you. Be your own Dreamweaver!

6. **Visit your Inner Child** - If you still haven't locked your "where I go from here" plan, give yourself permission to take on the task from the point of view of your younger self. Close your eyes and envision yourself as a seven-year-old, before school and the world trained you into limitations. What did that child want

to be when he/she grew up? What did they do for fun? Imagine yourself looking into those innocent eyes and asking them what you should do next, and don't self-edit what comes to you. Your inner child knows you better than your adult self ever will.

7. **Say it forward** – Affirm your confidence in your future by affirming your gratitude in advance. Say thank you to the universe in your knowingness for everything that is already coming to you. By offering our highest loving energy to our future self, we are doing more than imagining what is to come, we are amplifying the energy that will put us in alignment to manifest it.

8. **Role Play** – Whether real, or imaginary, asking for help from idols or entrepreneurs in the field in which you wish to play, is a great bliss amplifier. Study and replicate the lives and actions of people who have followed their imaginations and are doing what you want to do. Try that role on for size.

9. **Bling Out Your Bliss** – Remember that bliss is where every dream begins...you have the power to amplify yours, and create anything you wish. Albert Einstein once said, "Logic will get you from "A" to "B". Imagination will take you everywhere." Disney's imagination took him from one animated cartoon to the conglomerate of international amusement parks, animation studios and a global media empire. Think of every celebrity you know... any artist, sports hero, musician, actor, writer, designer, chef, explorer, teacher, builder...the list goes on and on for where we can amplify our bliss.

10. **Practice Surrender** – When you are able to let go of all expectations, this is where you will find your purpose. It will land on your shoulder like a butterfly on a summer day, full of delightful surprise at finding you at the right place, at exactly the right time. This is where life becomes "better than you have imagined," because there is no place for disappointment in a stagnant outcome. You will instead be living your version of "happily ever after," because this is of course, is your storybook that you have written. In surrendering to your own story, you will find your bliss.

Making your Bliss Your Vacation or Your Vocation:

Know that you know the tools for exploring and activating your bliss, you have the choice of how to apply it to your lifemap. There are two ways of mapping your bliss to your life: Make it your vocation or make it your vacation.

Making bliss your vacation:

You may find that hiking in the mountains is your bliss. You love nothing more than getting up early on a brisk spring morning and heading out on a quiet trail through the woods and drinking in the clean, fresh air because it feeds your soul. But you are a single mother of 3 children, living in New York City. It doesn't mean that you need to quit your job, leave your family and become a park ranger (although you could). It might just mean that to balance out your "have-to's" you have to add to your "want-to's." Part of it is just saying, "Hey bliss, I know what you are. I have a bliss wish living and growing inside of me, and

I'm going to shine light on and water that bliss. And over time, I will give that bliss more of my attention. But for now, I'm doing what I have to do until I can get there.

Giving yourself the time to nurture that longing is an enriching way to follow your bliss. It gives it a seat at the table. You can grow it one tiny project, one tiny action, one directional step at a time. And over time, if it is truly meant to be part of your purpose, it will find a way to live in your world. It must...it's one of the laws of the universe!

Making bliss your vocation:

If you are ready to take the big step in making your bliss your vocation, know this doesn't need to be a big leap off a grand cliff and done all at once. You can become the boss of your bliss and do it in tiny steps to help you get your footing. There is wisdom in the saying "Walk before your run." Use the tools above to help you map the first lap of your journey, until you are comfortable with the knowingness that it is the route you want to be on both professionally and financially.

Through the chapters in this book, there are countless stories of seekers just like you who have found their purpose and their vocation in the same place. But it is by feeling out those smaller steps and gathering the affirmations of the inner knowing that you are in the right place that will ultimately show you where to land.

Trust yourself, and trust that you will be shown the way by following both this inner and outer guidance from your internal GPS and by using your 4 "I's"– Inspiration, Intuition, Intention, and Imagination.

Bliss + Fear = Breakthrough

Ki is one of the best Bliss Activators that I know and has made her personal version of bliss her vocation. She is a great example of someone who really lived out all three phases of her own Bliss-topia... and like most of us, she never really knew it..until she faced her biggest fear.

Writing a book about it.

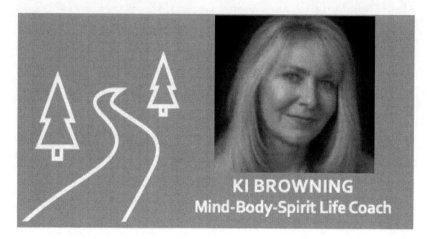

KI BROWNING
Mind-Body-Spirit Life Coach

Ki's Story

I've spent most of my life studying and teaching about healing practices. As a Mind-Body-Spirit Life Coach, I've spent over 20 years in the health and wellness field, researching unique ways to cultivate a purposeful, productive and peaceful life. In my twenties, I had an opportunity to travel the world, and visited over 30 countries and US cities. During my pilgrimage to India, I visited and meditated in ancient caves and temples. I climbed the Himalayan Mountains, and participated in silent retreats at Buddhist Monasteries in Thailand.

I dedicated my life to learning everything I could about mediation, Reiki, dreams, past-life regression, nutrition, and yoga. It sounds like a long list, doesn't it? But as I began working with my clients and fellow seekers, I noticed that my travels and my own learnings along the way could help others.

My joy is being able to share this knowledge in a way that is simple, in bite sized nuggets that everyone can try on for size, in the way that best suits their lives and their lifestyles. When I wrote and published my book, *Zenergy*, it began with the idea of sharing these methods and practices. But in the process, I learned so much about myself. It caused me to really think through all the things I struggled with along the way.

Through my work and life experiences, I have come to believe that when we are born there is a plan, Great Spirit's plan. We arrive in a specific region of the world to parents of a particular race, faith, and socioeconomic status. We intend to meet certain people at specific times, possibly marry and maybe have children. We explore the world, develop our careers, find ways to contribute and learn many lessons. Some people make lifelong decisions from something that happened in kindergarten or elementary school and live that notion for 80 years. Many will never question what was said to them by an absent-minded teacher or a distracted parent; they just believe one person's opinion and live it. One whole lifetime can be surmised into that one sentence if we let it. Don't get stuck believing what you, as a child or a teenager, assumed to be true.

You can create a new sentence at any age or any stage... don't waste the rest of your days in a daze. Consider creating an empowering inspiring sentence with a joyous viewpoint and an exciting trajectory. Find activities that generate an enthusiastic spirit! It's better to fulfil your life purpose sloppily than to fulfil someone else's purpose successfully. Get ready to hop on that joy train and take off into the

heavenly stargate to the next dimension, the next reality."
(Zenergy p.309 - 310)

Walking in Blissful Awareness

Ki's book has been so successful that the Dr. Deepak Chopra
Center endorsed her book, and she delivered a presentation
to Chopra Certified Instructors ("training the trainers"). If
you enjoyed the samplings from the "blissful bestie's" section above, I'd encourage you to sample Ki's *Zenergy* book
for what I like to call "a spiritual buffet" of soul nourishing
practices and information that will help you further explore
methods and tools for cultivating your mind, body and spirit.

Paving Your Road Forward

As we have learned, our biggest lessons can be reflected in
both our "love" as well as in our "fear" milestones.

While you many easily see how bliss highlights the "Love"
impulses in your heart, we have also identified how purpose
can shine through from the deepest darkest crevasses of
pain. This is where fear, shame, despair and anger live and
hide. It loves to burrow deep, with heavy, dense roots that
threaten to suffocate us with its forceful power to block
out all light and love.

*Then when looking back at your life, you will see that
the moments which seemed to be great failures followed
by wreckage were the incidents that shaped the life you
have now. You'll see that this is really true. Nothing can
happen to you that is not positive. Even though it looks
and feels at the moment like a negative crisis, it is not.*

*The crises throws you back and when you are required
to exhibit strength, it comes."*

—Joseph Campbell.

But as we have learned...these fear milestones are our greatest teachers. They are not just the things that have happened to us. They are the things that happen *for* us.

It can take time, but if we can get to a place where we can see these experiences as blessings, as the gift that they are, we can then flip this into our purpose for what we teach others.

We've already read many examples of those people in this book.

These are not stories of celebrities, corporate leaders or gurus. These are real people taking potentially life-crippling experiences and turning them from sorrow to purpose. This is truly what it means to embrace our humanness and have the courage rise up out of the ashes and shine the light on the path to make it easier for those to follow. It is their gift, their journey from fear to love, that becomes blissful blessings for us all.

Walking the Walk Down Lifemapping Lane

Since teaming up with my friend Robyn, my perception of my life's mission has continued to evolve. Following our work on the Oprah project, we worked together to create a vision for a television show that we believe will provide breakthrough programming that will help wake people up by giving them a makeover for their soul. And, within that vision, we've mapped out a platform for creating an even larger global platform that offers all of the things in my original network idea, but on an even bigger scale.

But we are also committed to living within the practice of being open to everything and attached to nothing. And in doing so, we continue to follow wherever our inspiration leads us. This year, we launched a YouTube channel and podcast, that celebrates our story as seekers, while also exploring the spiritual modalities and teachings that have inspired us. We have no idea where these conversations will take us, but we know that doing this work together is part of our life's work. It's putting it out to the universe that we are open and willing vessels to communicate what we know as the collective voice of our souls. And we recognize that our separate life journeys have given us the perfect experiences and complimentary skills to create and elevate this work together.

Where the road will lead, we have no idea. But we are content in our now. We listen and act on our inspiration. We will let the universe pave the road in front of us, blissfully content that we are living out our souls' purpose, by helping others find theirs.

I have learned so much from Wayne Dyers writings about all of the "bliss factors" that I've talked about in this book, and most specifically within this chapter. For me, this speaks so well about all I've learned concerning my own 4 "I's" which Wayne shared in this final chapter of his last book, "I Can See Clearly Now." It's as if this was the final thought that he really wanted to leave us with.

As I look back on my life, it's not a far stretch for me to conclude that there is some kind of a plan that is always at work. Nor is it unreasonable to conclude that this plan is being directed by the same force that keeps the planets aligned, opens the buds of all of the flowers, and gives life to all manners of creation here and everywhere else in the universe. I now pay much closer attention to what shows up for me and I'm willing to listen carefully to any inclination I might have and act accordingly, even if it leads me into unknown territory. I encourage you to do the same.

Examine the major turning points in your life and look carefully at all of the so-called coincidences that had to arise in order for you to shift direction. At that moment, you took it as a coincidence, you had a free will and you made a choice.

At that same moment there was something much bigger than you, something that you are always connected to that was also at play. That "something" was setting up the details so that you could fulfill the purpose you signed up for from when you made the leap from Spirit to form – from nowhere to now here.

The teachers are always there. Your degree of readiness to pay attention and listen carefully to your highest self, and act on what your intuitive self tells you, enlivens your awareness of your teachers. Sharpen your insight and be willing to trust that what you are feeling inside is what you should be doing, regardless of what everything and everyone around you might be saying to the contrary."

So well said Wayne.

Remember, it's ok to drive in the slow lane

What is it they say, "life is the journey, not the destination?" It is all but a constant unfolding, that truly never ends, and certainly not in one lifetime. If you have gotten this far in my book, I know you are eager to manifest this next part of your journey. I promise you, if you use even just a few of these tools you've practiced in these last few chapters, I know you will find what direction you need to go. I must also say with love, that "following" and not forcing the flow of your journey is as important as the "finding."

All of this really is just life...a school for learning. And it's not about the lesson, but the opportunity to learn. Life is really meant to be a buffet...a sampling of all of flavors of experiences and emotions, which would quickly get boring if you ate the same meal over and over again. Savor each sample, create your own plate, with the flavors and textures that fit you.

This is not about finding it all in a day. It is truly a journey. So, make yours a joy-ride.

Feel free to re-write your story, any time you choose.

OK, here's the last thing I want to tell you. You can always rewrite your past history. I didn't want to mention that when we were going through our mapping exercise, because, well, what would the fun have been in that? I mean, look at everything you've learned about yourself.

But the truth is, from this point on, now that you understand who you are and how you got here, not one of the things from your past has to impact another moment of your future. In fact, now that you can bless all of those experiences, knowing that you signed up for them and planned for them to take place, you can release their power over you. Since you now know your purpose and have been through your life review, you can decide exactly what you want to do from here.

So, what's it going to be?

The only sure thing in life is that it will continue to change. As much as we'd all love to pave the way forward on our Lifemapping road, the truth is that there are always things that come in our way to throw us off course.

Always, always, please be gentle on yourself. Try as best you can to drift with the flow, even when the pace of the water rises, threatening to throw you underwater. This still continues to be my favorite exercise for working my way forward on my LifeMap. Remember you always have the power to change the outcome of your movie. So, when the great things happen...celebrate like it's nobody's business. When you make mistakes, love that main character with all the compassion and understanding that you know your audience would. Never judge yourself because we are all just doing the best we can.

Remember the words of the great ancient poet Rumi to help you always affirm your personal motto of greatness. I am always inspired by these words that transcend time.

> *You were born with potential*
> *You were born with goodness and trust*
> *You were born with ideals and dreams*
> *You were born with greatness*
> *You were born with wings.*
> *You were not meant for crawling, so don't.*
> *You have wings.*
> *Learn to use them and fly.*

> —Rumi

You are now and forever always will be enough. You are now and always will be in charge of your own story.

 SOUL GOODY BAG

Here are some resources mentioned in this chapter for you for further exploration:

- **Zenergy Mind Body Spirit—by Ki Browning Zenergize**
  Your Mind-Body-Spirit! This comprehensive reference book provides the discovery tools of time tested,

scientifically proven methods to help you traverse these challenging and changing times. Whether nutrition, meditation, yoga, self-discipline, emotional balance, spiritual development or understanding your Divine Life Purpose, you will find ways to stay balanced. The path to wellness just got a little easier with Ki's rich knowledge at your fingertips

- *Wishes Fulfilled: Mastering the Art of Manifesting by Dr. Wayne W. Dyer.* The greatest gift you have been given is the gift of your imagination. Wishes Fulfilled is designed to take you on a voyage of discovery, wherein you can begin to tap into the amazing manifesting powers that you possess within you and create a life in which all that you imagine for yourself becomes a present fact.

- *Inspiration, Your Ultimate Calling* by Dr. Wayne Dyer There's a voice in the universe calling each of us to remember our purpose—our reason for being here now, in this world of impermanence. The voice whispers, shouts, and sings to us that this experience of being in form, in space and time, knowing life and death, has meaning. The voice is that of inspiration, which is within each and every one of us. Each chapter in this book is filled with specifics for living an inspired life. From a very personal viewpoint, Wayne Dyer offers a blueprint through the world of spirit to inspiration, your ultimate calling.

- *The Power of Intention: Learning to Co-Create Your World, Your Way by Dr. Wayne Dyer.* This book explores intention— as something you do— as an energy you're a part of. We're all intended here through the invisible power of intention. This is the first book to look at intention as a field of energy that you can access to begin co-creating your life with the power of intention.

- *Developing Intuition* by **Shakti Gawain.** In Developing Intuition, Shakti Gawain offers simple, practical lessons that will teach you how to get in touch with your intuition, learn to recognize its various forms, and process the intuitive knowledge that comes your way. You'll develop a deeper connection to the soul level of your existence and bring a new understanding to your daily life.

- *Daring Greatly: How the Courage to be Vulnerable Transforms the Way we Live, Love, Parent and Lead* by **Brene Brown.** Every day we experience the uncertainty, risks, and emotional exposure that defines what it means to be vulnerable or to dare greatly. Based on twelve years of pioneering research, Brené Brown PhD, LMSW, dispels the cultural myth that vulnerability is weakness and argues that it is, in truth, our most accurate measure of courage.

- *Awaken the Spirit Within* by **Rebecca Rosen.** With a unique and refreshing blend of self-help, wisdom, and spiritual insight, Rebecca Rosen helps us "wake up" and start living our lives with divine intention and purpose offering inspired and invigorating ideas to give our lives clarity and deeper meaning.

- ***Dream Sight: A Dictionary and Guide for Interpreting Any Dream* by Dr. Michael Lennox** Combining warmth and a touch of irreverence, *Dream Sight* is both a unique teaching tool and a fun reference guide that gives you everything you need to understand your dreams and your innermost self. This educational resource, features an alphabetized list of over 300 dream symbols and images with classic meanings.

- ***Spirit Almanac – A Modern Guide to Ancient Self Care* by Emma Loewe and Lindsay Kellner.** *The Spirt Almanac* provides readers with potent, accessible rituals they will want to call on again and again throughout the year to feel more grounded, aligned with their purpose, and in touch with their own innate sense of knowing.

- ***Zenergy Mind Body Spirit* by Ki Browning -** Zenergize Your Mind-Body-Spirit! This comprehensive reference book provides the discovery tools of time-tested, scientifically proven methods to help you traverse these challenging and changing times. Whether nutrition, meditation, yoga, self-discipline, emotional balance, spiritual development or understanding your Divine Life Purpose, you will find ways to stay balanced. Restore peace, joy and understanding to your life today! Join Ki as she takes you on a journey of the Mind, Body and Spirit, empowering you through Zenergy Boosts, recipes, yoga poses and exercises to complete at your own pace. The path to wellness just got a little easier with Ki's rich knowledge at your fingertips.

AFTERWORD

WHERE DO WE GO FROM HERE?

As it turned out, I ended up writing most of this book, sitting in the parking lot of my local library. Every night, I'd jump in my car and navigate my way through mostly deserted streets to my designated spot with the view of the park, watching the sun set from the cocoon of my car. It was my space of dedicated quiet to have conversations with myself. It provided a place for my thoughts to think without expectation; quiet time to exhale and breathe to let my heart and soul listen to itself.

I loved every minute of this be-ing with myself...and you.

As I edit these final chapters, the world is slowly coming out of a global pandemic. Here in NJ where I live, the "shelter in place" rules are still being enforced, requiring social distancing and the wearing of facial masks in public spaces.

An odd time to write about coming out of ourselves, when we are being told to hide.

It has been a surreal time in America, that I could never have imagined back in December 2019, when my work on this book began. I thought this would all be just a fun experiment, a challenge to myself, and a way to explore how deep the Lifemapping concept could go that would help with my workshops and coaching sessions.

After years of riding trains, and an endless commute to my office In Manhattan, I was one that relished the opportunity to work from home. And then to escape down the road inside my little "office on wheels," for my daily download of inspiration, parked across from a peach orchard coming into spring blossoms.

One night I had been working late there in that library parking lot, and I was startled by a flashlight and a knock on my car passenger window. A local police officer was on patrol, and was checking in to be sure I was ok. I laughed and explained that I had been "pent up" in my house with three males (husband, son and dog) and needed a quiet place to reflect and write my book in peace, and that he would be seeing a lot of me here.

"We're getting a lot of that," he said.

"Makes sense," I thought.

Everyone was starting to need a place to escape the escape. But I was committed to not taking this opportunity for granted, not for a minute. The planet was giving permission for all of us to have a "time out" and give our lives a think.

And so, it is with you, dear friend. No matter when this comes into your hands, I hope this book, this time, this experience, collectively has offered you the opportunity to take a time out for yourself.

Each milestone of your life, each experience and each day offers you an opportunity to reassess and re-examine your life **at a point in time.** It doesn't have to be a global event, or a catastrophe, to draw your attention, because all of it matters- every tiny piece of it.

You chose this time specifically for this life experience. And you are doing what you came in to do. The key is to KNOW that you are DOING IT and that every choice, like living through this pandemic, is about love or fear.

And I say that with total love and respect for everyone who has lost a loved one. Everyone who has lost a job, or a business or relationship because of this outbreak. Everyone who has had their school or prom, or wedding or baby shower cancelled. Everyone who is reading this wondering how to recover from their post traumatic fear or not knowing quite what to do next.

All of this still applies.

And if you don't know where to go from here, please reach out to me here karen loenser Lifemapping. I have a dedicated place on my website where you can share your story or send me a direct email. You'll find links to my down-loadable workbooks, and information about my ongoing workshops for both individual and small groups who want more or personalized sessions for developing their own customized Lifemaps.

Sometimes, all you need is an interpreter. And that's what I'm here for.

When I began writing in December 2019, I wasn't sure that I had anything to say. I wasn't even sure that my Lifemapping concept was worthy of a book. But as the winter months unfolded, the world succumbed to a global pandemic that changed, well...everything.

As this world health crisis unfolded, so too did my drive like so many, to find my own personal meaning in life. If there was one question that I asked myself over and over during this time, it was **what was this here to teach me** and what was I supposed to do with that lesson? If the world and I got through all of this, and nothing changed, what a waste it would be.

So, if not now when? How much more time was I willing to lose?

I am thankful that I personally had no close friends or family members who were lost, but the effects came close enough to feel the profound impact of how fragile life can be...how fast the normal can change.

And like you, I want my contribution to this planet to be real....to be as I intended.

As I finish these final thoughts, ironically, the sun is setting over the library parking lot. It's Mother's Day, and spring has thankfully, finally arrived. Families are huddled on carefully spaced blankets over on the park grass...the blue-sky crisp with fluffy clouds. The genuine-ness of this moment is sweet. It's a sunny imprint in time. I am fulfilled and filled with joy for me and for you.

And as if on cue, the band REM sends love from the car radio.

"It's the end of the world as we know it, and I feel fine."
XOXO

ABOUT DEFINING MOMENTS PRESS

Built for aspiring authors who are looking to share trans-formative ideas with others throughout the world, Defining Moments Press offers life coaches, healers, business pro-fessionals, and other non-fiction or self-help authors a comprehensive solution to get their book published without breaking the bank or taking years.

Defining Moments Press prides itself on bringing read-ers and authors together to find tools and solutions for everyday problems.

As an alternative to self-publishing or signing with a major publishing house we offer full profits to our authors, low-priced author copies, and simple contract terms.

Most authors get stuck trying to navigate the technical end of publishing. The comprehensive publishing services offered by Defining Moments Press mean that your book will be designed by an experienced graphic artist, available in printed, hard copy format, and coded for all eBook readers, including the Kindle, iPad, Nook, and more.

We handle all of the technical aspects of your book creation so you can spend more time focusing on your business that makes a difference for other people.

Defining Moments Press founder, publisher, and #1 bestselling author Melanie Warner has over 20 years of experience as a writer, publisher, master life coach, and accomplished entrepreneur.

You can learn more about Warner's innovative approach to self- publishing or take advantage of free trainings and education at: MyDefiningMoments.com

Defining Moments Book Publishing

If you're like many authors, you have wanted to write a book for a long time, maybe you have even started a book...but somehow, as hard as you have tried to make your book a priority, other things keep getting in the way.

Some authors have fears about their ability to write or whether or not anyone will value what they write or buy their book. For others, the challenge is making the time to write their book or having accountability to finish it.

It's not just finding the time and confidence to write that is an obstacle. Most authors get overwhelmed with the logistics of finding an editor, finding a support team, hiring an experienced designer, and figuring out all the technicalities of writing, publishing, marketing, and launching a book. Others have actually written a book and might have even published it but did not find a way to make it profitable.

For more information on how to participate in our next Defining Moments Author Training program, visit: www.MyDefiningMoments.com. Or you can email melanie@MyDefiningMoments.com.

OTHER BOOKS BY DEFINING MOMENTS™ PRESS

- *Defining Moments: Coping With the Loss of a Child -* by Melanie Warner https://www.amazon.com/dp/B07X2FGPCJ

- *Write your Bestselling Book in 8 Weeks or Less and Make a Profit - Even if No One Has Ever Heard of You -* by Melanie Warner

- *Become Brilliant: Roadmap From Fear to Courage* – by Shiran Cohen https://www.amazon.com/Become-Brilliant-Roadmap-Fear-Courage-ebook/dp/B089R64Q8B

- *Rise, Fight, Love, Repeat: Ignite Your Morning Fire -* by Jeff Wickersham https://www.amazon.com/dp/B08CY5S21P

- *Life Mapping: Decoding the Blueprint of Your Soul -* by Karen Loenser

- *Ravens and Rainbows: A Mother-Daughter Story of Grit, Courage and Love After Death –* by L. Grey and Vanessa Lynn https://www.amazon.com/dp/B08BZYWLCQ

- *Pivot You! 6 Powerful Steps to Thriving During Uncertain Times –* by Suzanne R. Sibilla https://www.amazon.com/dp/B08DL28784

- *A Workforce Inspired: Tools to Manage Negativity and Support a Toxic-Free Workplace –* by Dolores Neira. https://www.amazon.com/Workforce-INSPIRED-Negativity-Toxic-Free-Workplace- ebook/dp/B08F-2H95KM/

- *Friendship Choices -* by Benedictta Apraku

- *Journey of 1000 Miles -* by Hank DeBruin and Tanya McCready

Some authors have fears about their ability to write or whether or not anyone will value what they write or buy their book. For others, the challenge is making the time to write their book or having accountability to finish it.

It's not just finding the time and confidence to write that is an obstacle. Most authors get overwhelmed with the logistics of finding an editor, finding a support team, hiring an experienced designer, and figuring out all the technical-ities of writing, publishing, marketing and launching a book. Others have actually written a book and might have even published it, but did not find a way to make it profitable.

For more information on how to participate in our next Defining Moments Author Training program visit: www. MyDefiningMoments.com. Or you can email melanie@ MyDefiningMoments.com